STUDYING FOR PHARMACOLOGY QUESTIONS ON NCLEX

OVERVIEW

Pharmacology on NCLEX is primarily related to common drugs, common drug uses, and safety measures necessary when using pharmacologic agents. Typically, there are questions over a standard few drugs, and typically there are one or two questions over drugs that are not commonly used. The questions related to uncommonly used drugs are generally about safety measures related to all drugs and the nursing graduate is able to determine the correct answer to the question, many times, even if the student is not familiar with the drug in question. Understanding some basic concepts about pharmacology, reviewing a select few drugs, and knowing how to monitor for problems with drugs given will enable most students to do well on answering pharmacology questions on the NCLEX.

WHAT TO STUDY ABOUT PHARMACOLOGY:
* Classes of drugs
* Generic drug name clues
* Side effects of certain drugs
* Basic pharmacology safety principles

WHAT <u>NOT</u> TO STUDY RELATED TO PHARMACOLGY:
* Brand/propietory names of drugs
* Most drug dosages
* Most individual drugs
* A list of drugs, rather than conditions

HOW TO STUDY FOR PHARMACOLOGY QUESTIONS:
* Identify the conditions most commonly treated with medications
* Know the desired effect of pharmacologic agents for different conditions
* Identify key drugs to know by body system (included in this book)
* Learn to classify many drugs by recognizing the ending letters (the suffixes)
* Review differences in drug effects in pediatric and geriatric clients
* Make flash cards to remember drug groups, common drugs, side effects

PRINCIPLES OF PHARMACOLOGY

<u>Route of Administration</u>
* In order for the drug to work, it must be delivered to the target tissue
* The route of administration affects how long it takes the drug to get to the target area

* Usual routes of administration include topical(by skin or mucous membranes), oral(by mouth), parenteral(by injection), and intravenous(by vein)

Topical Route of Administration
* In the topical route, drugs are quickly absorbed and there are fewer side effects because the drugs are put on the tissue where they are quickly absorbed. Frequently the drug is placed on the tissue that is affected by some condition and it works to alter the condition.
* Suppositories are another example of the topical route. Absorption is through the mucous membranes and the stomach and liver are bypassed allowing for rapid absorption. Anti-nausea drugs and fever reducers are often given per rectum.
* Examples of topical agents include eye drops, ear drops, lotions/creams/ointments, and suppositories

Oral Route of Administration
* In the oral route, the drug must first be absorbed through the stomach, then pass through the liver, and then go through the bloodstream to the correct area in the body. When the drug passes through the liver, that is called the first pass effect. The amount of drug available to the body may be greatly reduced due to the first pass effect of the liver filtering the drug.
* Drugs taken orally may be absorbed slowly if there is decreased gastrointestinal motility, altered pH in the stomach, or problems with the liver.

Parenteral Route of Administration
* The parenteral route bypasses the liver and the drug is absorbed by blood passing through the tissue in which the drug is deposited. This includes drugs administered in muscle, subcutaneous tissue, or the intradermal skin layer.
* Small amounts of drugs to be rapidly absorbed may be given with a 1/2 inch needle in subcutaneous tissue. Examples include heparin and insulin
* Skin testing for inflammatory response is given intradermally. This includes allergy testing and TB skin tests.
* Intramuscular injections:Large amounts of drugs should be given in muscle. In drugs intended for intramuscular injection, drug distribution may be altered if the drug is delivered to fat rather than muscle or if there is little muscle mass. In most adults IM injections require use of a 1.5 inch needle.

Intravenous Administration
* The intravenous route is the quickest means for delivering medication as it goes directly in the bloodstream.
* The risk to the patient may be greater with this route due to the quick absorption of the drug.
 * The nurse should be cautious to instill IV drugs at the rate in which they are ordered to avoid bad side effects.

Drug Excretion
* Most drugs are excreted through the kidneys. Altered kidney function may lead to drug toxicity.
 * The "half-life" of a drug refers to how quickly the drug is excreted. A long half-life means the drug stays in the body a long time. Drugs with the initials SR(sustained release), XL, DR or described as slow or sustained release stay in the body for a long time. Drugs given once a day generally have a longer half life than drugs given more frequently.
 * When measuring the metabolism of a drug, the onset of action, peak action, and duration of action are considered.

Monitoring Drug Therapy
 * Determining the maximal concentration and effectiveness of a drug may be done by measuring peak and trough levels, or the levels when the drug is at its highest and lowest levels. These levels may be measured when using certain antibiotics.
 * When monitoring drug therapy the nurse should monitor the patient's condition, and whether therapeutic drug levels have been attained. If the drug reduces the patient's symptoms and does not cause significant side effects it is generally considered an effective drug for the patient.
* Drug levels are usually monitored on drugs that have a high risk for causing serious side effects if drug toxicity occurs. These drugs include digoxin, theophylline, phenotoin (dilantin)/other seizure medications, and lithium. Drug levels may be monitored when other drugs are used, but these are the most common drugs in which levels are routinely monitored.
* The effectiveness of warfarin (Coumadin) and heparin are commonly measured by measuring the PT/PTT or INR.

Drugs and Pediatric
 * Pediatric drugs are usually dosed on a mg/kg of body weight basis.
 * Children are at greater risk for drug toxicity because of lower renal function than that of older persons, increased body water, and smaller range of dosages.

Drugs and Geriatric Patients

    * Older persons (geriatric) may be at risk for drug toxicity due to poor kidney function, dehydration, poor absorption in the stomach and gut, and poor filtration through the liver.

    * Renal function is best measured by measuring creatinine clearance through a 24 hour urine collection.

    * In general, geriatric dosing should be started at 1/2 adult dosing and should be increased very gradually. The rule is "start low and go slow".

    * Polypharmacy refers to being on multiple medications at one time. The more medications the patient takes, the greater the risk of a drug reaction. Patients who take 5 or more medications at one time are at 100% risk for a drug reaction.

SPECIAL DRUG ADMINISTRATION TIPS:

* Always observe the 5 rights when giving medications:

Right patient (check arm band)

Right drug (check medication record and medication)

Right time (check medication record)

Right route (check medication record)

Right dosage (check medication record)

* Eye drops should be instilled in lower lid (conjunctival sac) being cautious not to touch the dropper tip to the eyelid surface. Oinments are often easier to use than drops.

 * Ear drops are instilled by straightening the ear canal and filling it with the drops. The patient needs to lie on the opposite side for 5-10 minutes after administration to allow for absorption of the drops, or the drops will run out.

* Nose drops should be instilled with the patient in a position with the head tilted back. Drops are instilled toward the midline. The patient should remain supine for 5 minutes and should avoid blowing his nose afterwards.

* When giving medications by nasogastric the nurse should check for placement first. When giving NG meds or meds by gastric tube, the tubing should be flushed with water before and after giving the medication.

DRUG CLASSIFICATION:

Drugs are generally classified by their mechanism of action and by their mechanism of action and by the target function they serve.

They are also classified by the body system for which they exert their major influence.

1. The physician orders a loading dose of 350 mg of aminophylline for a respiratory client. The medication comes in ampules of 250 mg in 10 mL of fluid. How many mLs should the client receive?

   A.   8 mL
   B.   14 mL
   C.   16 mL
   D.   20 mL

2. What is aminophylline's primary action?

   A.   Increases heart rate and contraction
   B.   Promotes pulmonary circulation
   C.   Relaxes smooth muscles in the bronchioles
   D.   Stimulates the receptors in the brain stem

3. Choose the medication that best provides immediate treatment for a client experiencing rapid atrial fibrillation.

   A.   Lidocaine IV push
   B.   Digoxin (Lanoxin) 0.25 mg IV now
   C.   Atropine 0.05 mg IV
   D.   Propranolol (Inderal) 35 mg PO

1.
Answer: B
Rationale: Ordered/
                Desired ÷ dose on hand x solution

$$\frac{350}{250} \times 10 = 14$$

Body System: Respiratory

2.
Answer: C
Rationale: Medication is used for clients with respiratory problems, i.e. bronchiole constriction. Aminophylline is indicated for treatment of respiratory problems.

Body System: Respiratory

3.
Answer: B
Rationale: Lanoxin will slow the rate and convert the atrial fibrillation to a sinus rhythm in some individuals.

Body System: Cardiovascular

1.   **Select the body structure that produces naturally occurring steroids.**

      A.   Anterior pituitary
      B.   Adrenal medulla
      C.   Posterior pituitary
      D.   Adrenal cortex

2.   **Mineralocorticoids are primarily responsible for the regulation of which body function?**

      A.   Carbohydrate and protein metabolism
      B.   Secondary sexual development
      C.   Electrolyte and fluid balance
      D.   Function of the cardiovascular system

3.   **An accident victim is admitted to the ICU for observation and a possible skull fracture. The physician has ordered dexamethasone (Decadron) 4 mg q6h to be given IV. Why is this medication being given to this client?**

      A.   Suppresses the immune response and therefore will prevent infections from the injury
      B.   Reduces the swelling of the brain and prevents increased intracranial pressure
      C.   Disrupts the formation of histamine and will prevent allergic reactions to medications
      D.   Increases protein and carbohydrate metabolism so that healing of injured tissues will occur at an increased rate

1.
Answer: D
Rationale: The adrenal cortex manufactures these hormones, particularly cortisol and aldosterone.

Body System: Cardiovascular

2.
Answer: C
Rationale: The "mineralo" of mineralocorticoids refers to minerals (Na, K, Cl, Mg, etc.) and H_2O.

Body System: Endocrine

3.
Answer: B
Rationale: One of the major effects of steroid medications is to reduce inflammation and swelling.

Body System: Endocrine

1. A 16-year-old client comes into the emergency room covered from head to toe with a red raised rash which is being scratched vigorously. Two days ago he had been on a camping trip and was exposed to poison oak. A diagnosis of contact dermatitis is made and the physician writes a prescription for hydrocortisone (Cortef) 10 mg PO each morning for 14 days. What is the most important teaching measure that the nurse needs to convey to this client?

   A. Take the medication on an empty stomach because food inactivates it
   B. Skip doses if the client feels lightheaded
   C. Watch for symptoms of respiratory depression
   D. Make sure the medication is taken with food or milk

2. The physician orders methylprednisolone (Solu-Medrol) 350 mg IV now. The medication comes from the pharmacy labeled 500 mg per 4 mL. How much of this medication will the nurse have to give?

   A. .35 mL
   B. 3.5 mL
   C. 2.8 mL
   D. .28 mL

1.
Answer: D
Rationale: Steroid medications are very irritating to the stomach and may lead to gastritis or ulcers if taken on an empty stomach.

Body System: Endocrine

2.
Answer: C
Rationale: Math - 500 : 4 :: 350: x

$$500x = 4 \times 350 \text{ or } 1400$$
$$x = \frac{1400}{500}$$

$\underline{\text{Desired dose}}$
on hand strength x solution

$$x = 2.8 \text{ mL}$$

Body System: Endocrine

1. **Select the most important nursing consideration when administering IV methylprednisotone (Solu-Medrol) to a client.**

    A. Give only as an IV bolus or push medication
    B. Dilute the medication in 50 cc D_5W and give over 30 minutes IV piggyback (IVPB) to prevent thrombophlebitis
    C. Give the medication only through a central line IV to prevent irritation of the veins
    D. Give the medication within 30 minutes of mixing

2. **Which statement will verify to the nurse that teaching has been successful concerning the use of oral corticosteroid?**

    A. "I need to take these on an empty stomach so they will work quickly."
    B. "I need to refill this prescription so I can avoid stopping this medication suddenly."
    C. "I need to check my blood pressure every day to see if it is dropping."
    D. "When I feel better, I can stop taking these pills."

3. **A client is admitted to the hospital exhibiting an exacerbation of symptoms of systemic lupus erythematosus. Identify an important factor the nurse will need to consider when educating the client about taking prednisone.**

    A. Client's increased susceptibility to infections
    B. Client's depression and suicidal tendencies
    C. Client's need for extra glucose and fluids
    D. Client's tendency to excrete potassium and sodium

1.
Answer: A
Rationale: The medication is most effective when given IV push.

Body System: Endocrine

2.
Answer: B
Rationale: Suddenly stopping steroid medications can produce serious side effects including Addison's Crisis.

Body System: Endocrine

3.
Answer: A
Rationale: Major side effect of corticosteroids is immune system depression.

Body System: Immune System

1.   **A 22-year-old client has been taking high doses of prednisone (Deltasone) for recently diagnosed systemic lupus erythematosus (SLE) and is beginning to develop Cushing's syndrome. What are some of the key symptoms the nurse would observe which are indicative of this syndrome?**

      A.   Urinary frequency, excessive thirst and low blood pressure
      B.   Slow heart rate, cold intolerance and dry skin
      C.   Moon face, buffalo hump and hirsutism
      D.   Dry mouth, tachycardia and blurred vision

2.   **Select the most severe short-term side effects of oral glucocorticoid medications.**

      A.   Peptic ulcers and GI bleeding
      B.   Hypoglycemia and CNS stimulation
      C.   Delayed wound healing and immunosuppression
      D.   Increased appetite and muscle wasting

3.   **Select the statement that best defines thyroid stimulating hormones.**

      A.   Thyroid hormones are made in the anterior pituitary
      B. T_4 (Thyroxine) is more active than T_3 (triiodothyronine)
      C.   Thyroid hormones only affect the heart and muscles
      D. T_3 (triidothyronine) is more active than T_4 (Thyroxine)

1.
Answer: C
Rationale: These medications cause abnormal fat distribution and fluid retention.

Body System: Endocrine

2.
Answer: A
Rationale: These medications are very irritating to the stomach.

Body System: Endocrine

3.
Answer: D
Rationale: T_4 is converted by the body to T_3.

Body System: Endocrine

1.   **Levothyroxine (Synthroid) is a synthetic form of which of the thyroid hormones?**

     A.   Thyrocalcitonin
     B.   Triiodothyronine
     C.   Thyroxine
     D.   Thyrotropin-releasing hormone

2.   **Identify side effects a client may experience while taking levothyroxine   (Synthroid)**

     A.   Nervousness, tachycardia and tremors
     B.   Somnolence, bradycardia and paresthesia
     C.   Hyperglycemia, hypertension and edema
     D.   Buffalo hump, constipation and sodium loss

3.   **A client diagnosed as having hyperthyroidism, is taking propylthiouracil (Propyl-Thyracil). Identify the primary action of propylthinouracil.**

     A.   Destroys part of the thyroid gland so that it will not produce as much thyroid hormone
     B.   Inhibits the conversion of T_4 to T_3
     C.   Suppresses the anterior pituitary gland to slow down its hormonal secretions
     D.   Sedates the CNS and suppress cardiac function

1.
Answer: C
Rationale: Thyroxine (T_4) has a synthetic form.

Body System: Endocrine

2.
Answer: A
Rationale: Thyroid hormones stimulate the metabolic, cardiac and nervous systems.

Body System: Endocrine

3.
Answer: B
Rationale: This medication prevents the conversion of the inactive T_4 to the more active T_3.

Body System: Endocrine

1.   **A client with hyperthyroidism is started on propylthiouracil (Propyl-Thyracil). Select the statement by the client that indicates client teaching has been effective.**

      A.   "I realize it may take a few weeks before this medication becomes effective."

      B.   "Taking aspirin will help the medication work more effectively"

      C.   "I must avoid all activities where I can get cut."

      D.   "I must take this medication with food or antacids."

2.   **Select the statement that best describes the primary mode of action for insulin.**

      A.   Insulin allows cells to absorb and use glucose

      B.   Insulin increases the stores of fat and glycogen

      C.   Insulin is made in the alpha cells of the pancreas

      D.   Insulin increases fat and protein metabolism

3.   **The physician orders an IV of D5 1/2 NS to start at 200 mL per hour on a diabetic client. An initial dose of 10 units of insulin is given IV. What type of insulin is used?**

      A.   NPH insulin

      B.   Lente insulin

      C.   Ultralente insulin

      D.   Regular insulin

1.
Answer: A
Rationale: The body must use up all the circulating T_3 before effects can be seen.

Body System: Endocrine

2.
Answer: A
Rationale: This is how insulin works in the body.

Body System: Endocrine

3.
Answer: D
Rationale: Regular insulin is the only insulin that can be given IV because it is in a pure form.

Body System: Endocrine

1.   **Which medical condition would require a 54-year-old client to receive captopril (Capoten)?**

      A.   Chronic hypertension
      B.   Venous thrombosis
      C.   Hypertensive crisis
      D.   Unstable angina pectoris

2.   **Choose the description that refers to bacterial organisms that are no longer destroyed by the usual types and amounts of antibiotics.**

      A.   Nosocomial infective organisms
      B.   Indigenous flora bacteria
      C.   Resistant bacterial organisms
      D.   Opportunistic organisms

1.
Answer: A
Rationale: This is an ACE inhibitor commonly used for chronic hypertension.

Body System: Cardivascular

2.
Answer: C
Rationale: Bacteria become resistant and requires larger doses or different antibiotics.

Body System: Antibiotic

1.   **Select the primary mode of action for the penicillin class of antibiotics.**

   A.   Interferes with DNA production in the cell
   B.   Inhibits cell wall synthesis
   C.   Destroys messenger RNA
   D.   Bacteriostatic against gram-negative organisms

2.   **The physician orders amoxicillin (Amoxil) 500 mg IVPB q8h for an adult client with an upper respiratory tract infection. What is an appropriate nursing action in relation to this medication?**
   A.   Question the order because the route of administration is incorrect
   B.   Give the medication as ordered
   C.   Question the order because the dose is too large
   D.   Question the order because the medication does not work against the organisms that cause respiratory infections

3.   **What is the most important nursing measure to consider before giving a penicillin class medication IVPB to a client for the first time?**

   A.   Double check the dose and route of the medication
   B.   Give the client a subcutaneous injection of epinephrine
   C.   Ask client if he/she has a history of allergy to penicillin
   D.   Give the medication within two hours of mixing and on an empty stomach

1.
Answer: B
Rationale: Penicillin prevents the production of an enzyme that maintains the integrity of the bacteria cell wall. The wall ruptures and the bacteria die.

Body System: Antibiotics

2.
Answer: A
Rationale: This medication is only given orally.

Body System: Antibiotics

3.
Answer: C
Rationale: Many clients have allergies to penicillin medications. Giving penicillin by IV can cause anaphylaxis.

Body System: Antibiotics

1. **Identify the class of medications that have a similar mode of action to cephalosporins.**

    A.   Aminoglycocides
    B.   Penicillins
    C.   Tetracyclines
    D.   Antituberculin medications

2. **A 22-month-old child is diagnosed with a UTI (urinary tract infection) and the physician prescribes oral cefaclor (Ceclor). How should the nurse instruct the mother to administer the medication?**

    A.   Concurrently with meals to prevent GI irritation
    B.   Immediately after the child has eaten
    C.   One hour before or two hours after a meal
    D.   30 minutes before or after a meal

3. **A mother administers the cefaclor (Ceclor) appropriately to her 22-month-old child. The UTI clears but the mother notes patches of "milk" in the child's mouth that she can not remove. The child is very fussy when eating. Which condition would the nurse expect to find after examination?**

    A.   A superinfection with Candida albicans
    B.   Allergic reaction to the medication manifested by the development of stomatitis
    C.   A herpes simplex virus (Type I) post antibiotic therapy
    D.   An idiosyncratic reaction to the medication

1.
Answer: B
Rationale: Both groups inhibit cell wall synthesis.

Body System: Antibiotic

2.
Answer: C
Rationale: The medication works best on an empty stomach.

Body System: Antibiotic

3.
Answer: A
Rationale: Candida infections are a common side effect of antibiotic therapy.

Body System: Antibiotic

1.   A 21-year-old client has been taking cephalexin (Keflex) 500 mg
      tid PO for an infected cut on the arm. On the eighth day of a
      10-day course of treatment, the client begins experiencing nausea,
      bloating, diarrhea and generalized GI discomfort. What is the
      most probable reason for these symptoms?

      A.   The development of gastric ulcers secondary to the
            medication
      B.   The dosage of the medication is too large
      C.   An allergic reaction to the medication
      D.   Alterations in the normal flora of the GI tract secondary to
            the effect of the medication

2.   Which organisms are effectively treated by using the
      aminoglycosides?

      A.   Upper respiratory tract infections
      B.   Gram-negative organisms
      C.   Gram-positive organisms
      D.   Urinary tract infections

3.   The physician orders gentamicin (Garamycin) 65 mg IVPB now.
      The medication comes from the pharmacy labeled 80 mg in 2 mL.
      How much will the nurse draw up for administration?

      A.   .8 mL
      B.   1.2 mL
      C.   1.625 mL
      D.   16.2 mL

1.
Answer: D
Rationale: The antibiotic has killed many of the bacteria normally found in the GI tract of the client.

Body System: Antibiotic

2.
Answer: B
Rationale: Gram-negative organisms are difficult to destroy with the penicillins and cephalosporins.

Body System: Antibiotic

3.
Answer: C
Rationale: Math - 80: 2 :: 65 : x

$$80x = 130$$

$$x = \frac{130}{80}$$

$$x = 1.625$$

Body System: Antibiotic

1.   **Which physical response is considered the most serious side effect of the aminoglycosides?**

    A.   Ototoxicity
    B.   Photosensitivity
    C.   Syncope
    D.   Nephrotoxicity

2.   **A 32-year-old client has a severe URI (upper respiratory infection.) The nurse teaches the client about the respiratory system's defense mechanisms against microbial invasion. Choose the statement that most accurately describes the ciliated mucus membrane function of the respiratory system's defense mechanisms.**

    A.   Small hair-like structures in the bronchioles trap small particles and move them toward the trachea with a wave-like motion
    B.   The goblet cells and bronchial glands in the lower respiratory tract secrete mucus that traps other particles
    C.   Peristaltic waves sweep mucus from the lower respiratory tract toward the pharynx where it is swallowed or expectorated
    D.   The IgA antibodies and lysozyme in the saliva break down bacterial cell walls

3.   **Which medication is the most useful for treating meningitis or brain abscesses?**

    A.   Chloramphenicol   (Chloromyetin)
    B.   Gentamicin   (Garamycin)
    C.   Ampicillin   (Omnipen)
    D.   Ceftazidime   (Fortaz)

1.
Answer: D
Rationale: Renal failure and death can result from the use of these medications.

Body System: Antibiotics

2.
Answer: A
Rationale: The cilia are small hairs that trap particles that bypass the upper airway filtering mechanisms.

Body System: Respiratory

3.
Answer: A
Rationale: This is one of the few antibiotics that will cross the blood-brain barrier.

Body System: Neurology

1. A client develops a UTI. The physician prescribes sulfamethoxa-zole/ trimethoprim (Bactrim DS) 500 mg bid PO for 10 days. What important element is to be included in the instructions for this client?

   A. Drink 2,000 to 3,000 mL of water per day and stay out of direct sunlight
   B. Monitor weight daily for renal failure
   C. Avoid sexual activity until the infection clears
   D. Stop taking the medication when burning on urination goes away

2. A 64-year-old client has been exposed to pulmonary tuberculosis. PPD skin test has converted from non-reactive to reactive indicating that the client has developed some antibodies to the bacteria. The client has no other symptoms. Assuming that there are no contraindications, which medication will most likely be prescribed for prophylaxis of this disease?

   A. Streptomycin
   B. Chloramphenicol (Chloromycetin)
   C. Isoniazid (INH)
   D. Metronidazole (Flagyl)

3. A client who has contacted TB often forgets to take the medications and subsequently develops active pulmonary tuberculosis. The client's medication is changed to rifampin (Rifandin) and isoniazid (INH) daily, PO. What is the rationale for using two medications?

   A. The incidence of allergic reactions is reduced when the two medications are used simultaneously.
   B. Even if the client forgets to take one of the medications, the other will be effective.
   C. The two medications have a synergistic effect when given together and quickly destroy the organism.
   D. The TB bacillus quickly becomes resistant to the one medication when it is used alone but is less likely to become resistant if two medications are used.

1.
Answer: A
Rationale: An increase in fluid intake should be part of the regimen for all oral antibiotic therapy, and even more so in the case of a UTI.

Body System:Antibiotics

2.
Answer: C
Rationale: Isoniazid is the most common medication used to treat potential TB clients.

Body System: Respiratory

3.
Answer: D
Rationale: One difficulty in treating TB is its tendency to become resistant. Combining antibiotics will help prevent this.

Body System: Respiratory

1. What is the primary reason for administering pyridoxine (Vit. B6) concurrently with INH?

    A. Decreases dysfunction
    B. Peripheral neuritis
    C. Ototoxicity
    D. Damage to visual acuity and color vision

2. Which medical history would be a contraindication to the client's use of isoniazid (INH) and/or rifampin (Rifadin)?

    A. Hepatitis
    B. Cardiovascular disease
    C. Allergy to aspirin or seafood
    D. Childhood tuberculosis

3. A 92-year-old client is admitted to the hospital with a complaint of "feeling sick", a temperature of 103.8°F, dehydration and a serious urinary tract infection. The client is placed on bedrest and started on metronidazole (Flagyl) 1,000 mg q8h IVPB. What is the most likely reason that the client is receiving this medication?

    A. An infection with a protozoa organism
    B. Allergic to other antimicrobial infections
    C. A systemic infection with an aerobic organism
    D. This medication has fewer side effects and causes less damage to the kidneys than other medications

1.
Answer: B
Rationale: The numbness and tingling associated with use of INH can be lessened by pyridoxine.

<u>Body System: Respiratory</u>

2.
Answer: A
Rationale: These medications are very toxic to the liver and any type of liver disease would prevent their use.

<u>Body System: Respiratory</u>

3.
Answer: C
Rationale: Although this medication is an antifungal, it also works well against systemic active organisms as indicated by the client's symptoms.

<u>Body System: Antibiotics</u>

1. The physician usually prescribes a loading dose of theophylline (in the form of aminophylline) based on the client's ideal body weight. For a particular client, the physician bases the loading dose on the actual body weight, which is less than ideal body weight. Why would the lower weight be used as the determining factor?

    A.   Using the lower weight prevents theophylline intolerance
    B.   Using the lower weight helps prevent toxicity
    C.   Using the lower weight increases the medication's half-life
    D.   Using the lower weight yields optimal serum concentration levels of 5 to 10 mcg/mL

2. How does aminophylline and the other brochodilators affect the cardio-vascular system?

    A.   Increases the renal blood flow and glomerular filtration rate, which improves cardiac function
    B.   Decreases the force and rate of myocardial contractions by depressing the myocardium
    C.   Constricts the systemic blood vessels by causing tension in the vascular smooth muscles
    D.   Causes excessive cardiac stimulation that can lead to renal failure

1.
Answer: B
Rationale: It is likely that in using the ideal weight, the client would receive too much medication.

Body System: Respiratory

2.
Answer: A
Rationale: They have a positive inotropic effect on the heart and blood vessels, thereby increasing cardiac output.

Body System: Respiratory

1. **In planning care for a client with schizophrenia, the nurse recognizes that all antipsychotic medications are derivatives of phenothiazine. How do antipsychotic medications differ from each other?**

    A.   Degree of sedation manifested
    B.   Potential to cause tardive dyskinesia
    C.   Potency and side effect
    D.   Method of administration

2. **A physician orders guaifenesin (Robitussin) for a client diagnosed as having bronchitis. Choose the appropriate client-teaching points the nurse should stress with this client.**

    A.   Avoid becoming pregnant during guaifenesin therapy
    B.   Tell other physicians about the guaifenesin therapy; it could alter thyroid function test results
    C.   Drink 2 to 3 liters of fluid per day to thin and loosen respiratory secretions
    D.   Never take the medication on an empty stomach

3. **A client is on IV Heparin, 5500 units q4h. A PTT is drawn a half hour before the 0800 dose. The results come back at 0755 with the PTT at 110 seconds (Control at 20 seconds). What is the most appropriate action for the nurse to take?**

    A.   Give the next dose, since it is near the time to be given
    B.   Immediately check the client's vital signs and LOC
    C.   Call the lab to redraw the sample, since an error must have been made
    D.   Hold the dose and call the results to the physician

1.
Answer: C
Rationale: Phenothiazines are similar to chlorpromazine, the prototype, but differ from it in potency and degree of side effects.

Body System: Psychology

2.
Answer: C
Rationale: Good hydration is always an important element in the care of clients with lung disease.

Body System: Respiratory

3.
Answer: D
Rationale: This PTT is much greater than would be considered therapeutic. The physician needs the PTT results so a lower dose of heparin can be ordered.

Body System: Cardiovascular

1.   **Before administering a phenothiazine to a client, choose the response that best determines the choice of medication for treatment.**

    A.   Client's general response to pharmacotherapy

    B.   Capacity to decrease psychotic symptoms with a minimum of side effects

    C.   Capacity to decrease target symptoms regardless of side effects

    D.   Degree of side effects caused by treatment

2.   **A 51-year-old heavy smoker has a nonproductive cough that leaves the client totally exhausted. The physician prescribes codeine, 20 mg PO q4h. How does codeine compare with dextromethorphan as an antitussive?**

    A.   Dextromethorphan is not as effective as codeine

    B.   Dextromethorphan is more addictive than codeine

    C.   Dextromethorphan and codeine have similar analgesic properties

    D.   Dextromethorphan has a greater CNS depressant effect than codeine

3.   **If a heavy cigarette smoker is debilitated, why would the physician not prescribe a narcotic antitussive?**

    A.   It could increase respiratory secretions, placing the client at risk for developing pneumonia

    B.   It could make the client particularly susceptible to hypersensitivity reactions

    C.   It could precipitate an asthmatic attack

    D.   It could increase secretion viscosity and suppress the cough reflex

1.
Answer: B
Rationale: Since all phenothiazines are similar, choice is based on client response to medications that decrease psychotic (or target) symptoms with the fewest side effects.

Body System: Psychology

2.
Answer: B
Rationale: Codeine is a narcotic medication and is considered a controlled substance due to its addiction potential.

Body System: Respiratory

3.
Answer: D
Rationale: The cough reflex is already suppressed in debilitated clients, and narcotic medications would only suppress it further.

Body System: Respiratory

1.   **A client complains of chest pain. What is the first action the nurse initiates before giving the client the first nitrate dose?**

    A.   Take pulse, blood pressure, then administer an IV nitrate
    B.   Take pulse, blood pressure, then administer transdermal nitrate
    C.   Administer sublingual nitrate immediately, check pulse and blood pressure
    D.   Assess the degree, type and location of the pain before administering the nitrate

2.   **A client with a history of cardiac disease complains of chest pain. As the nurse prepares to administer nitrate sublingually, the client complains of a dry mouth. What should the nurse do first?**

    A.   Give the client the sublingual nitrate followed by sips of water
    B.   Give the client sips of water followed by the sublingual nitrate
    C.   Give the client the sublingual nitrate, then offer a glass of water
    D.   Do not give the sublingual nitrate and notify the physician

3.   **A 71-year-old client takes a beta-adrenergic blocker for angina. While visiting this client, the community health nurse notes that the apical pulse rate is 54 beats per minute. What should the nurse do?**

    A.   Tell the client to stop taking the medication, then reassess the pulse rate the next day
    B.   Tell the client to stop taking the medication and to discuss it with the physician during the next weekly appointment
    C.   Contact the client's physician to prescribe tapering of the medication
    D.   Instruct the client to continue the medication as prescribed

1.
Answer: D
Rationale: The assessment must verify that the chest pain is due to cardiac disease before using NTG.

Body System: Cardiovascular

2.
Answer: B
Rationale: If the oral mucous membranes are dry, the NTG will absorb slowly or not at all.

Body System: Cardiovascular

3.
Answer: C
Rationale: A slow pulse rate may be a sign of toxicity for this medication. Only the physician can change the dosage.

Body System: Cardiovascular

1. A 48-year-old client takes diltiazem (Cardizem), a calcium channel blocker. When should the client have the medication "held" and the physician be notified?

    A. The physician order is for 40 mg PO qid
    B. Client is hospitalized with liver failure
    C. Pulse rate is 84 beats/minute
    D. Blood pressure is 102/70 mm Hg

2. What is the most common contraindication for the use of nitrates in clients with angina?

    A. History of GI bleeding
    B. History of severe hypertension
    C. History of increased intracranial pressure
    D. History of pulmonary embolism

3. A client is to take chlorpromazine (Thorazine) at home for a psychotic condition. What information should be explained to the client and the significant other regarding this medication?

    A. Stools may be black
    B. Stools may be white
    C. Urine may be reddish-brown
    D. Urine may be greenish

1.
Answer: B
Rationale: The calcium channel blockers are metabolized in the liver
and can be very toxic in the presence of liver failure.

Body System: Cardiovascular

2.
Answer: C
Rationale: The vasodilation effect of nitrates will increase the
intracranial pressure even more.

Body System: Cardiovascular

3.
Answer: C
Rationale: Although it may turn the urine pink to reddish-brown, this is
not harmful.

Body System: Psychology

1.   **What action should clients avoid when taking sympatholytic agents for hypertension?**

      A.   Eating foods high in potassium
      B.   Suddenly stop taking the medication
      C.   Changing position gradually
      D.   Decreasing fluid intake

2.   **Identify the medication that, when taken with heparin, will increase the client's tendency to bleed.**

      A.   Aspirin
      B.   Oral contraceptives
      C.   Penicillin
      D.   Antihistamines

3.   **A history of which medical condition would be a contraindication for a client to receive a PO or IV anticoagulant?**

      A.   Cardiovascular disease
      B.   Acute depression
      C.   Thrombocytopenia
      D.   Diabetes mellitus

1.
Answer: B
Rationale: If these medications are suddenly stopped, they can cause a rebound effect that may lead to MI or hypertensive crisis.

Body System: Cardiovascular

2.
Answer: A
Rationale: Aspirin coats the platelets so that they will not clump, thus acting as an anticoagulant.

Body System: Cardiovascular

3.
Answer: C
Rationale: This is a disorder in which the platelet count is low, thus causing the client to bleed excessively, even without anticoagulants.

Body System: Cardiovascular

1.   A 27-year-old client has allergies to grass and dust. The physician
     prescribes diphenhydramine (Benadryl) PO for this condition.
     What is the normal dosage range for this medication?

     A.   5 to 15 mg PO qd
     B.   15 to 20 mg PO bid
     C.   25 to 50 mg PO tid
     D.   100 to 300 mg PO qid

2.   Promethazine HCL (Phenergan) is classified as an antihistamine.
     Select another common use for this medication.

     A.   Relief of anxiety
     B.   Relief of nausea
     C.   Prevention of edema during surgery
     D.   Relief of urinary retention during pregnancy

3.   A physician writes an order for promethazine (Phenergan), 500
     mg IM to be given now and q4h for a client. Based on your knowl-
     edge of this medication, what should be done first by the nurse?

     A.   Give the medication as ordered because it is a normal dose
     B.   Hold the medication because it should be given PO only
     C.   Hold the medication and check the dosage with the
           physician
     D.   Give only half the dose now and see what effects it has
           before giving the rest

1.
Answer: C
Rationale: This is the normal range for an adult.

Body System:Respiratory

2.
Answer: B
Rationale: Commonly given IV or IM for nausea postoperatively.

Body System: Gastrointestinal

3.
Answer: C
Rationale: The correct dosage range for this medication is 25 mg to 50 mg.

Body System: Gastrointestinal

1.   **What is the primary use for isorbide (Isordil)?**

    A.   Relief of allergies to foods and medications
    B.   Relief of chronic anginal pain
    C.   Dilation of the bronchials in asthma
    D.   Stimulation of the cardiac muscles

2.   **What is the normal adult dose for isorbide (Isordil)?**

    A.   10 mg PO q4h
    B.   150 mg SL q2h PRN
    C.   25 to 50 mg IM q6h
    D.   100 to 150 mg IM q12h

3.   **Select the most important nursing measure in relationship to a client who is taking isorbide (Isordil)?**

    A.   To monitor respiratory status 30 minutes after administration
    B.   To give the medication with food or milk
    C.   To monitor blood pressure after administration
    D.   To monitor for bronchodilation after administration

1.
Answer: B
Rationale: This medication is a long-acting form of NTG and is used for chest pain and sometimes BP control.

Body System: Cardiovascular

2.
Answer: A
Rationale: This is the normal dose.

Body System: Cardiovascular

3.
Answer: C
Rationale: Like most nitrates, this medication may lower blood pressure.

Body System: Cardiovascular

1.   A 54-year-old client is receiving methylodopa (Aldomet) for
        chronic hypertension. Choose the mode of action for this
        medication.

        A.   To inhibit the conversion of angiotensin I to angiotensin II
        B.   Blockage of the alpha-1 receptors
        C.   Direct dilation of the arteries and veins
        D.   Blockage of the beta-1 receptors

2.   A client is receiving phenytoin (Dilantin) for seizures and the
        physician orders chlorpromazine (Thorazine) as a neuroleptic
        medication. What would the nurse expect the physician to do?

        A.   Monitor serum levels of phenytoin
        B.   Decrease the dosage of phenytoin
        C.   Monitor serum levels of Thorazine
        D.   Taper the client off phenytoin

3.   Select the medical condition that is primarily treated with
        mannitol (Osmitrol).

        A.   Hypertensive crisis
        B.   Congestive heart failure
        C.   Head injuries
        D.   Pulmonary edema

1.
Answer: B
Rationale: It blocks the stimulation of the alpha-1 receptors, thereby producing vasodilation.

Body System: Cardiovascular

2.
Answer: A
Rationale: Thorazine inhibits phenytoin metabolism, so it could cause phenytoin toxicity. Also, phenothiazine medications lower the seizure potential in clients.

Body System: Neurology

3.
Answer: C
Rationale: Mannitol is a hypertonic solution that pulls fluid from swollen brain tissues, thereby reducing intracranial pressure.

Body System: Neurology

1. A client who is being started on chlorpromazine asks the nurse: "Why do I need to take this medication?" Choose the nurse's best explanation.

    A.   "To help you organize your thoughts."
    B.   "To keep you from having nightmares."
    C.   "It will help you to sleep."
    D.   "It will decrease depression."

2. What is the most important nursing measure to consider before administering mannitol (Osmitrol) to a client?

    A.   Make sure the bottle is free of crystals
    B.   Give the medication with a full glass of water
    C.   Use a syringe large enough to give the medication in one injection
    D.   Make sure the client is sitting or lying down

3. A 78-year-old client is admitted with 4+ pitting edema of the legs and feet. The physician orders furosemide (Lasix) 35 mg IV for this client. The medication comes from the pharmacy labeled "40 mg/4 mL." How much of this medication will be administered by the nurse?

    A.   2.5 mL
    B.   3.5 mL
    C.   4.5 mL
    D.   5.5 mL

1.
Answer: A
Rationale: Antipsychotics are used in the treatment of acute and chronic psychoses, particularly when accompanied by increased psychomotor activity.

Body System: Neurology

2.
Answer: A
Rationale: Mannitol is a concentrated form of sugar and tends to crystallize when it stands for long periods of time or becomes cold.

Body System: Neurology

3.
Answer: B
Rationale: Math $40 : 4 :: 35 : x$

$$40x = 140$$
$$x = \frac{140}{40}$$
$$x = 3.5 \text{ mL}$$

Body System: Cardiovascular

1. **Choose the most important measure that the nurse should keep in mind when administering 3.5 mL of IV furosemide (Lasix).**

    A. Dilute it in 50 mL D$_5$W and give over 20 minutes
    B. Give it as rapidly as possible
    C. Give it only in normal saline
    D. Give it IV push over 3 to 4 minutes

2. **Choose the normal dosage range when administering heparin to an adult client.**

    A. 100 to 200 mg q 4 hours PO
    B. 2500 to 5000 units q 4 hours IV
    C. 125,000 to 500,000 units q 6 hours SC
    D. 500 to 1,000 q 4 hours IM

3. **A 23-year-old client who is taking birth control pills develops a thrombus in a leg. The client is admitted to the hospital and started on heparin. What is the most important nursing consideration for this client?**

    A. To monitor bleeding times with a PT
    B. Give aspirin for headaches and joint pain
    C. Hold all venipuncture for 5 minutes
    D. Have the client walk 4 hours to prevent pneumonia and joint stiffness

1.
Answer: D
Rationale: IV Lasix should be given no faster than 1 mL per minute.

Body System: Cardiovascular

2.
Answer: B
Rationale: This is the normal range.

Body System: Cardiovascular

3.
Answer: C
Rationale: Because of the anticoagulant effect, all venipuncture sites will tend to bleed unless pressure is applied.

Body System: Cardiovascular

1.   **Which statement by the client best indicates that the teaching instructions concerning heparin was successful?**

      A.   "This medication will dissolve the clots in my leg just like heparin."

      B.   "I need to eat lots of broccoli and cabbage in order to keep my strength up and recover completely."

      C.   "When I start feeling really good, I can stop taking this medication."

      D.   "I need to tell my dentist that I am taking this medication the next time I visit the office."

2.   **What is a normal dose of warfarin sodium (Coumadin) for a client suffering from a leg thrombus?**

      A.   7.5 mg qd

      B.   100 mg bid

      C.   2500 units qd

      D.   1 mg qid

3.   **Identify the primary mode of action of streptokinase (Streptase).**

      A.   Inhibits the adhesion of platelets

      B.   Interference of the synthesis of vitamin K in the liver

      C.   Breakdown of fibrin in clots

      D.   Prevents the conversion of thrombin to prothrombin

1.
Answer: D
Rationale: It is important to notify health-care providers before they perform any procedures that may cause bleeding.

Body System: Cardiovascular

2.
Answer: A
Rationale: The range is usually between 2.5 and 10 mg po.

Body System: Cardiovascular

3.
Answer: C
Rationale: The medication breaks down the protein in the collagenous fibers in clots.

Body System: Cardiovascular

1.   **Which medication can be used as an antidote for streptokinase (Streptase)?**

        A.   Protamine sulfate
        B.   Aminocaproic acid (Amicar)
        C.   Aquamephyton (vitamin K)
        D.   Atropine sulfate

2.   **Which condition may a client have who is taking naldolol (Corgard)?**

        A.   Hypertension
        B.   Peripheral edema
        C.   Increased intracranial pressure
        D.   Chronic bronchitis

3.   **What will client, who is started on dobutamine (Dobutrex), most likely experience?**

        A.   Hypertensive crisis
        B.   Unstable angina
        C.   Cardiogenic shock
        D.   Pulmonary embolus

1.
Answer: B
Rationale: Can also be used as an antidote for heparin.

Body System: Cardiovascular

2.
Answer: A
Rationale: This is a beta blocker that is used primarily for blood pressure control.

Body System: Cardiovascular

3.
Answer: C
Rationale: This is a positive inotropic medication used to increase the cardiac output.

Body System: Cardiovascular

1. **Butyrophenones, phenothiazines, haloperidol lactate, and thioxanthene belong to which group of medications?**

   A. Anxiolytics
   B. Antidepressants
   C. Anticholinergics
   D. Antipsychotics

2. **Which physical symptom is a side effect of prednisone (Deltasone) therapy?**

   A. Tinnitus
   B. Exfoliative dermatitis
   C. Glycosuria
   D. Nausea and vomiting

3. **Which precaution should the nurse advise the client of during teaching about prednisone (Deltasone)?**

   A. Take oral preparations of prednisone (Deltasone) before meals
   B. Never stop or change the amount of medication without medical advice
   C. Have periodic complete blood count while on the medication
   D. Wear sunglasses if exposed to bright light for an extended period of time

1.
Answer: D
Rationale: All of these are neuroleptic medications used to treat
psychotic conditions.

Body System: Neurology

2.
Answer: C
Rationale: Steroid medications increase the blood glucose and when it
gets high enough, it will spill into the urine.

Body System: Endocrine

3.
Answer: B
Rationale: Suddenly stopping steroid medications can produce rebound
steroid crisis.

Body System: Endocrine

1. **Which route of adminstration provides the most rapid absorption of medications?**

   A. **Sublingual**
   B **Subcutaneous**
   C. **Intramuscular**
   D. **Intravenous**

2. **In planning care for a client who is taking chlorpromazine (Thorazine), why should the nurse recognize that it is important to notify the physician and document signs and symptoms of tardive dyskinesia?**

   A. Tardive dyskinesia is always reversible
   B. Tardive dyskinesia is potentially irreversible
   C. The physician may increase the neuroleptic
   D. The physician will order an antidepressant

3. **Which potential complication of liver and/or kidney disease would be expected?**

   A. Unusual side effects of medications
   B. Allergic reactions to medications
   C. Medication interactions
   D. Cumulative or toxic effects of medications

1.
Answer: D
Rationale: Medications given IV become effective at the point of entry into the blood stream.

Body System: General

2.
Answer: B
Rationale: Early intervention to eliminate the medication at the first signs of tardive dyskinesia may cause the symptoms to remit if the medication is discontinued.

Body System: Psychology/Neurology

3.
Answer: D
Rationale: Decreased hepatic or renal function can lead to decreased excretion and toxicity.

Body System: General

1.   A 3-year-old client with asthma has oral medicines ordered. The
        nurse observes the mother saying to her child, "Here, Sally, take
        this candy - it is good. " as she give the child the medicine. What
        should the nurse do first?

        A.   Tell the client that she is endangering her child's life and
                that she should know better
        B.   Teach the mother not to equate medications with candy as a
                principle of poison control
        C.   Do nothing since Sally took the medicine — the result is
                what is important
        D.   Refuse to allow the mother to give the medicine again

2.   What is another term for adrenergic medications?

        A.   Sympathomimetic
        B.   Parasympathomimetic
        C.   Cholinergic
        D.   Anticholinergic

3.   A 55-year-old client who had been taking haloperidol (Haldol
        Decanoate) 100 mg for three years discontinues the medication.
        During the interview, the nurse notes that the client is blinking
        eyes continuously, with periodical tongue protrusion, and
        drooling. What is usually indicated by these assessments?

        A.   Neuroleptic-induced catatonia
        B.   Tardive dyskinesia
        C.   Dystonia
        D.   Akathisia

1.
Answer: B
Rationale: Children should be taught that medication is different from candy so that they will not take it by mistake.

Body System: General

2.
Answer: A
Rationale: These medications mimic the sympathetic nervous system.

Body System: General

3.
Answer: B
Rationale: Tardive dyskinesia is characterized by involuntary movements. If tardive dyskinesia is suspected, notify the physician at once. Movements may interfere with swallowing, breathing, gait, and result in falls.

Body System: Neurology

1.   After receiving albuterol mini nebulized treatment for acute asthma for the first time, a client states, "I feel so nervous. Is something wrong?" What would be the best response by the nurse?

      A.   "The anxiety is probably related to your hypoxia."
      B.   "Are you allergic to anything?"
      C.   "You may be having an adverse over-reaction to the situation."
      D.   "Your heart beats faster while helping you breathe better."

2.   You are to give Atropine 0.6 mg to your client. The medication comes gr. 1/150 per mL. How many mL's should be administered?

      A.   .5 mL
      B.   1 mL
      C.   1.5 mL
      D.   2 mL

3.   Aminophylline 250 mg in 500 cc D_5W is ordered at a rate of 30 cc/hour. How many mg's are being delivered per hour?

      A.   10 mg
      B.   15 mg
      C.   20 mg
      D.   25 mg

1.
Answer: D
Rationale: This is true and is a therapeutic response.

Body System: Respiratory

2.
Answer: C
Rationale: Math: grain $1/150 = 0.4$ mg
$0.4 : 1 :: 0.6 : x$
$0.4x = 0.6$
$x = \dfrac{0.6}{0.4}$
$x = 1.5$ mL

Body System: Respiratory

3.
Answer: B
Rationale: Math: concentration = $\dfrac{250}{500}$

$= 0.5$ mg/mL

rate $= 0.5$ mg/mL x 30mL/hr
$= 15$ mg/hr

Body System: Respiratory

1. **Identify the one factor that makes digoxin (Lanoxin) a potentially lethal medication.**

   A.   Broad range for therapeutic effect; therefore, clients tend to "overtake" the medication

   B.   Effect on the liver and kidneys

   C.   Narrow margin of safety — toxic dose is close to therapeutic dose

   D.   Common usage among the elderly

2. **Identify the signs and symptoms present that would cause the nurse to withhold the medication and alert the physician while a client is receiving digoxin (Lanoxin).**

   A.   Dry mouth and/or postural hypotension

   B.   Tardive dyskinesia

   C.   Development of moon face and "buffalo hump"

   D.   Bradycardia and/or anorexia

3. **Which medical diagnosis is usually treated by giving NTG gr. 1/150?**

   A.   Cardiac dysrhythmias

   B.   Angina pectoris

   C.   Hypotension

   D.   Congestive heart failure

1.
Answer: C
Rationale: Therapeutic = 0.5 to 1.5 toxic = 2.

Body System: Cardiovascular

2.
Answer: D
Rationale: These are signs of Lanoxin toxicity.

Body System: Cardiovascular

3.
Answer: B
Rationale: NTG is used for this condition to dilate coronary arteries.

Body System: Cardiovascular

1. The nitroglycerin bottle is labeled: "NTG 0.4 mg per tablet". A client is receiving NTG grains 1:150. What dosage should the client be instructed to take?

    A.   One tablet per dose
    B.   One and one-half per dose
    C.   Two tablets per dose
    D.   Three tablets per dose

2. Furosemide (Lasix) 40 mg IV push has been ordered as a "stat" dose for a client who is in acute congestive heart failure. The medication vial states 10 mg per mL. Which method should the nurse use when administering this IV medication?

    A.   Over a one-minute period
    B.   Over a four-minute period
    C.   As fast as the nurse can push it in, as speed is of importance
    D.   In 50 mL D₅W, and slowly let it drip into the vein

3. If a medication is known to cause ototoxicity, which nursing action is appropriate to implement before starting therapy with this medication?

    A.   Obtain a BUN and creatinine clearance test
    B.   Obtain a thorough visual assessment of the client
    C.   Assessment of the first cranial nerve
    D.   Obtain a baseline audiogram

1.
Answer: A
Rationale: Math: 1 grain = 60 mg

$$\frac{60}{150} = 0.4 = 1 \text{ tablet}$$

Body System: Cardiovascular

2.
Answer: B
Rationale: Math: 10 : 1 :: 40 : x

$$10x = 40$$
$$x = \frac{40}{10}$$
$$x = 4 \text{ mL given 1 mL/min}$$

Body System: Cardiovascular

3.
Answer: D
Rationale: Ototoxicity damages the eighth cranial nerve and may lead to hearing loss.

Body System: Cardiovascular

1. A client is taking (fluphenazine) Prolixin 0.5 mg qid. Which medication is given to control and/or prevent extrapyramidal signs and symptoms?

   A. Levodopa (Dopar) 0.5 mg qid
   B. Diazepam (Valium) 5 mg qid
   C. Methocarbamol (Robaxin) 1 g qid
   D. Benztropine (Cogentin) 2 mg qid

2. A client has developed a nosocomial infection with a gram-negative organism and has been placed on streptomycin. Choose the nursing action that would help prevent nephrotoxicity.

   A. Ask the physician to place the client on a diuretic
   B. Encourage fluids and keep an accurate I&O
   C. Encourage small, frequent feedings of high protein foods
   D. Maintain the client on a 2 gm (or less) sodium diet

3. Clients taking penicillin or other antibiotics often develop symptoms of nausea, "bloating", diarrhea, and cramping, etc. What is the usual cause for these symptoms?

   A. The development of gastric or duodenal ulcers secondary to the medication
   B. Milk intolerance related to the medication
   C. An allergic reaction to the medication
   D. Alterations in the normal flora of the GI tract secondary to the medication

1.
Answer: D
Rationale: Cogentin is an antiparkinsonian medication used to help prevent extrapyramidal signs and symptoms.

Body System: Neurology/Psychology

2.
Answer: B
Rationale: Fluids will help flush the medication from the body and prevent build up in the kidneys.

Body System: Antibiotics

3.
Answer: D
Rationale: The antibiotics kill the bacteria normally found in the intestines that helps in the digestion of food.

Body System: Antibiotics

1. **What is another name for "Pyridoxine"?**

   A. Vitamin B_{12}
   B. Vitamin B_6
   C. Vitamin multicomplex
   D. Purified vitamin B_1

2. **A few days after a client is started on antituberculin medication, the client makes a frantic call to the TB clinic and says, "My saliva and tears are red! What shall I do?" What is the best response by the nurse?**

   A. "This is a normal side effect of the medication. Don't be concerned, even though it does look alarming."
   B. "This is an indication that you are allergic to the medication. Stop taking it and come in to see the physician."
   C. "Have you been eating beets lately? That can cause your symptoms."
   D. "You sound concerned. You are wondering what to do about your red saliva and tears."

3. **A client is diagnosed as having idiopathic epilepsy and is taking phenytoin (Dilantin). Which instruction must the client understand completely?**

   A. Renal function studies are done approximately every other week
   B. Avoidance of the ingestion of CNS depressants such as alcohol or antidepressants
   C. Do not brush or floss teeth for fear of injuring the gums
   D. Swelling of the feet and ankles, although, a normal side effect of the medication

1.
Answer: B
Rationale: This is the other name for the medication.

Body System: Gastrointestinal

2.
Answer: A
Rationale: Information is true and good therapeutic communication technique.

Body System: Respiratory

3.
Answer: B
Rationale: This medication has a synergistic effect when mixed with other central nervous system medications.

Body System: Neurology

1.   **"Stomatitis" is a complication of several antineoplastic treatments including certain chemotherapeutic agents and radiation. What is affected by stomatitis?**

        A.   Lining of the stomach
        B.   The gastric mucosa
        C.   The esophagus
        D.   The oral cavity

2.   **Select the most appropriate lunch for a client with stomatitis.**

        A.   Crab salad, soft roll with butter, milk, vanilla ice cream
        B.   Fresh fruit cup, bowl of soup, crackers, tea
        C.   Cheese sandwich on French bread, carrot and celery stick, cup of soup, milk
        D.   Taco salad, corn chips, fresh fruit, tea

3.   **Which nursing measure is best to prevent the severe weight loss that is found in cancer clients with cachexia?**

        A.   Have family and friends remind the client to eat often
        B.   Vary dietary supplements and allow the client to choose
        C.   Offer high calorie finger foods frequently for snacks
        D.   Place a pitcher of juice or eggnog at the bedside

1.
Answer: D
Rationale: The mouth and gums are most often affected by stomatitis.

Body System: Chemotherapy

2.
Answer: A
Rationale: None of these foods would irritate the mucous membranes in the mouth.

Body System: Chemotherapy.

3.
Answer: C
Rationale: Frequent snacks will help the client maintain his or her normal weight.

Body System: Chemotherapy

1.   **Which substance, combined with alcohol, would be an appropriate example of a synergistic interaction between two substances?**

      A.   Aspirin
      B.   Tranquilizers
      C.   Antacids
      D.   Penicillin

2.   **Which nursing action is best to conduct before administering the first dose of meperidine (Demerol) to an elderly client with a fractured hip?**

      A.   Take vital signs
      B.   Place the client in restraints
      C.   Ask the client is there has ever been an addiction to narcotics
      D.   Ask if the client is addicted to alcoholic

3.   **When should meperidine (Demerol) be given to a client with a fractured hip in order to obtain best pain relief?**

      A.   Only after the pain has become quite severe in order to emphasize relief
      B.   Before the pain becomes severe
      C.   Every time the client asks for it
      D.   When you notice that blood pressure, pulse, and respirations are at least 20 above baseline

1.

Answer: B

Rationale: Synergism is an additive effect between two substances. Both of these have depressant effects on the central nervous system.

Body System: Analgesic

2.

Answer: A

Rationale: Need to assess the client's condition and vital signs to assess tolerance of the medication.

Body System: Analgesic

3.

Answer: B

Rationale: Pain medications are more effective if they are given before the pain reaches the severe level.

Body System: Analgesic

1.   A client with a fractured hip is to receive meperidine (Demerol) 75
      mg IM. Upon entering the room of this client, the nurse finds that
      the client's blood pressure is 110/74; pulse = 80, R = 16/minute.
      What should the nurse do on the basis of these findings?

      A.   Check the vital signs again in 15 minutes
      B.   Withhold the meperidine until checking with the physician
      C.   Administer a mild stimulant and then the meperidine
      D.   Give the meperidine as ordered

2.   A 68-year-old, Type II diabetic client, who is controlled by using
      oral hypoglycemics is admitted with pneumonia and respiratory
      distress. Blood sugar is 425, so the physician orders 10 units of
      regular insulin SC. The client questions the administration of the
      insulin because of the oral   hypoglycemics. What is the best
      response to the client's question?

      A.   "You have converted from Type II to Type I diabetes and
            will need insulin from now on."
      B.   "You are correct, I will question the physician before I give
            you this insulin."
      C.   "Don't worry about it, your physician knows what he is
            doing."
      D.   "Sometimes when people are very ill, they have to be on
            insulin for a short time."

3.   Select the most important action for a Type II diabetic on oral
      hypoglycemic medications?

      A.   Drink large quantities of fruit juice when taking medications
      B.   Eat on a regular schedule
      C.   Carry insulin and syringes in case of an emergency
      D.   Take medications with meals to prevent GI upset

1.
Answer: D
Rationale: These are normal vital signs and indicate that the client can have the medication.

Body System: Analgesic

2.
Answer: D
Rationale: The glucose tends to rise when clients are severely ill, but will return to normal when they recover.

Body System: Endocrine

3.
Answer: B
Rationale: This will prevent hypoglycemic reactions in these clients.

Body System: Endocrine

1.   **What is the primary effect of the mineralocorticoids on the body?**

        A.   Regulate carbohydrate and fat metabolism
        B.   Stimulate the sympathetic nervous system
        C.   Regulate electrolyte and fluid balance
        D.   Regulate growth of the sex organs

2.   **Select the primary mode of action of the glucocorticoids.**

        A.   Sodium excretion
        B.   Stimulate hypersensitive reactions
        C.   Increase antibody formation
        D.   Stabilize cell membranes

3.   **Select the best reason why glucocorticoids are often used in cases of head injury and CVA.**

        A.   They increase the heart rate
        B.   They reduce cerebral edema
        C.   They reduce the blood pressure
        D.   They increase the cranial capacity

1.
Answer: C
Rationale: They regulate Na, K, and H_2O.

Body System: Endocrine

2.
Answer: D
Rationale: These medications help stabilize the cell membranes and are used in most acute illnesses.

Body System: Endocrine

3.
Answer: B
Rationale: The anti-inflammatory effect reduces the swelling in the brain and intracranial pressure.

Body System: Endocrine

1.   **Select the most common side effect of long-term oral steroid use.**

        A.   Anemia
        B.   Bleeding tendencies
        C.   Peptic ulcers
        D.   Thick, tough skin

2.   **Which physical symptom indicates the development of Cushing's Syndrome in a client taking glucocorticoids?**

        A.   Moon face and hirsutism
        B.   Hair and weight loss
        C.   Moist, oily skin and hair
        D.   Dehydration and twitching

3.   **Identify an important nursing consideration for clients receiving steroid medications.**

        A.   Careful assessment for the signs of infection
        B.   Stop the medication immediately if any side effects develop
        C.   · Take the medication on an empty stomach to increase its absorption
        D.   Use the medications carefully in clients with pre-existing seizure

1.
Answer: C
Rationale: These medications are very irritating to the linings of the stomach and GI tract.

Body System: Endocrine

2.
Answer: A
Rationale: These symptoms are found in Cushing's Syndrome.

Body System: Endocrine

3.
Answer: A
Rationale: Because of the suppression of the immune system by these medications, infection is an ever-present problem.

Body System: Endocrine

1.   **What is the most severe and potentially lethal side effect of immunosuppressant medications?**

    A.   Hepatotoxicity
    B.   Tendency for organ rejection
    C.   Bone-marrow suppression
    D.   Gingival hyperplasia

2.   **Choose the most important element to include in a teaching plan for a client continuing medications after discharge from the hospital.**

    A.   Discuss refill schedule
    B.   Expected effects
    C.   Possible untoward reactions
    D.   Cost of the medication

3.   **Identify common side effects of the antineoplastic medications.**

    A.   Alopecia and cachexia
    B.   Hirsutism and acne
    C.   Hypovolemia and postural hypotension
    D.   Polycythemia and polyuria

1.
Answer: A
Rationale: Liver failure is a potentially lethal side effect of these medications.

Body System: General

2.
Answer: B
Rationale: The client should know what the medication is expected to do in relationship to the disease being treated.

Body System: General

3.
Answer: A
Rationale: Hair loss and severe weight loss are common side effects of most types of antineoplastic medications.

Body System: Chemotherapy

1. **Identify what nursing intervention will most help to reduce nausea that is often experienced by clients receiving chemotherapy.**

    A. Remove the cover from the food tray after bringing the tray into the client's room
    B. Offer the client spicy foods at frequent intervals
    C. Control odors in the client's environment
    D. Avoid sedating clients prior to treatment

2. **What should be the reply to the client if he or she decides that recommended chemotherapy has too many intolerable side effects, and elects to discontinue the therapy against medical advice?**

    A. Client must find another source of health care immediately
    B. There are two weeks to locate another source of health care
    C. The client is no longer eligible for assistance from the government
    D. Client may continue to use the oncology clinic for pain relief and/or palliative interventions

3. **A client is diagnosed as having acute, or narrow angle, glaucoma. What early symptoms might the nurse expect the client to display?**

    A. Blindness and colored spots in the visual fields
    B. Eye pain and "halos" around artificial lights
    C. Gradual swelling of the eyeball and eyelids
    D. Loss of central vision and visual acuity

1.

Answer: C

Rationale:　　　　Controlling odors, particularly ones that produce nausea, will help with this problem.

Body System: Chemotherapy

2.

Answer: D

Rationale:　　　　All clients have the right to refuse treatment at any time without punishment from the health care providers.

Body System: Chemotherapy

3.

Answer: B

Rationale:　　　　These are common early symptoms of this disorder.

Body System: Eye

1. The physician orders pilocarpine (Isopto Carpine) for a client's glaucoma condition. What is the classification of this medication?

    A.   Miotic
    B.   Diuretic
    C.   Mydriatic
    D.   Beta blocker

2. Another medication used to treat glaucoma is timolol maleate (Timoptic). How does this medication produces its effects?

    A.   Stimulates the cholinergic system
    B.   Causes increased secretion of sodium and water
    C.   Increases production of aqueous humor
    D.   Blocks the beta receptors of the autonomic system

3. What factor makes acetazolamide (Diamox) different from other medications used in the treatment of glaucoma?

    A.   Is administered directly into the eye
    B.   Can be taken systematically given intraocularly
    C.   Has very few side effects
    D.   Can be administered PO

1.
Answer: A
Rationale: This medication constricts the pupils causing a decrease in intraocular pressure.

Body System: Eye

2.
Answer: D
Rationale: The beta blockers reduce the production of aqueous humor, thereby reducing intraocular pressure.

Body System: Eye

3.
Answer: B
Rationale: This medication is a very powerful diuretic that is taken systematically rather than in eyedrop form.

Body System: Eye

1. The nurse is preparing a teaching plan for a client with schizo-phrenia and is taking fluphenazine decanoate (Prolixin). What is the medication's mode of action?

    A.   Increases the release of norepinephrine and serotonin available for binding sites
    B.   Blocks dopamine receptors in the brain and alter dopamine release and turnover
    C.   Prevents the reuptake of norepinephrine and serotonin by presynaptic neurons
    D.   Stimulates dopamine receptors

2. The physician orders chlordiazepoxide (Librium) every four hours as needed for a client detoxifying from alcohol. What is the most likely reason Librium was ordered?

    A.   Prevents nausea and vomiting from acute alcohol intoxication
    B.   Potentiates the effect of the alcohol so the client can drink less
    C.   Suppresses some of the symptoms of alcohol withdrawal
    D.   Keeps the client calm while en route to jail

3. Choose the most therapeutic dose of chlordiazepoxide (Librium) for a client in severe alcoholic withdrawal.

    A.   5 - 10 mg PO q hour PRN
    B.   50 - 100 mg IM q 4 hours PRN
    C.   250 - 500 mg IV q 2 hours PRN
    D.   30-60 mg IM q 12 hours PRN

1.
Answer: B
Rationale: Antipsychotic medications block receptor sites for the neurotransmitter dopamine in the brain and have a peripheral anticholinergic and alpha-adrenergic blockade effects.

Body System: Neurology/Psychology

2.
Answer: C
Rationale: This medication will help suppress the tremors and muscle cramping often seen in alcohol withdrawal.

Body System: Neurology/Psychology

3.
Answer: B
Rationale: This is a large dose of this medication but is required to control the symptoms of alcohol withdrawal.

Body System: Psychology

1.   A 68-year-old client is admitted to the hospital. While obtaining a history, the nurse discovers the client is receiving levodopa (Dopar). Identify the condition that would necessitate the use of levodopa.

    A.   Wide angle glaucoma
    B.   Hypertension
    C.   Type II diabetes
    D.   Parkinson's disease

2.   Select the most common use of orphenadrine citrate (Norflex).

    A.   Controls seizures in idiopathic seizure disorders
    B.   Prevents infections from gram + bacteria
    C.   For relief of pain from muscle spasm
    D.   As a back-up medication for the antitubercular medications

3.   What is a normal dosage range for digoxin (Lanoxin) in an adult with congestive heart failure?

    A.   5 - 10 mg PO bid
    B.   100 - 150 mg PO qd
    C.   15 - 25 grams PO q am
    D.   0.125 - 0.25 mg PO qd

1.
Answer: D
Rationale: This medication is one of the key medications used in Parkinson's and almost never used for any other condition.

Body System: Eye

2.
Answer: C
Rationale: This is a muscle relaxant used to relieve pain.

Body System: Musculoskeletal

3.
Answer: D
Rationale: This is a normal range and route for an adult.

Body System: Cardiovascular

1. **When the dose of a medication must be increased to get the same effect, choose the term that best describes the condition present.**

   A.   Tolerance
   B.   Physical dependence
   C.   Psychological dependence
   D.   Idiosyncratic reaction

2. **Which medication is most commonly used to treat attention deficit hyperactivity disorder (ADHD) or attention deficit disorder (ADD)?**

   A.   Dopamine (Intropine)
   B.   Oxazepam (Serax)
   C.   Methyphenidate (Ritalin)
   D.   Propylthiouracil (Propacil)

3. **Which adverse effect of dextroamphetamine sulfate (Dexedrine), or other stimulants used to treat attention deficit disorder (ADD), is best assessed by the parent's history of the child's progress?**

   A.   Cognitive functioning
   B.   Growth delays
   C.   Visual disturbances
   D.   Blood dyscrasias

1.
Answer: A
Rationale: As the body tissue become accustomed to a medication, it
will take larger and larger amounts to produce the same
effects, especially with CNS medications.

Body System: General

2.
Answer: C
Rationale: This medication appears to produce a chemical that these
children are lacking in their CNS.

Body System: Neurology

3.
Answer: B
Rationale: Stimulant medications used for treatment of attention deficit
disorder (ADD) can cause growth delays which are best
assessed by the child's parent or caretaker.

Body System: Neurology

1.   **Which condition would require a client to receive propranolol (Inderal)?**

   A.   Hypertension, migraine headache
   B.   Hyperthyroidism, hyperglycemia
   C.   Acute bronchitis, pneumonia
   D.   Cushing's Syndrome, Parkinson's disease

2.   **A 55-year-old client is admitted to the hospital and started on levothyroxine (Synthroid). What condition does this client likely have?**

   A.   Type I diabetes
   B.   Hyperthyroidism
   C.   Granulocytopenia
   D.   Hypothyroidism

3.   **A physician writes an order for a client to receive levothyroxine (Synthroid) 50 mg PO qd. What is the nurse's best response to this order?**

   A.   Hold the medication and check with the physician; the dose is too large
   B.   Give the medication as ordered and watch for side effects
   C.   Hold the medication and check with the physician; the dose is too small to be effective
   D.   Check the dosage with another nurse on the unit, and then give immediately

1.
Answer: A
Rationale: This medication is used to treat a wide variety of cardiovascular diseases due to its beta blocking MOA.

Body System: Cardiovascular

2.
Answer: D
Rationale: This medication is a synthetic form of thyroid hormone used to supplement low levels in the body.

Body System: Endocrine

3.
Answer: A
Rationale: The normal adult dose range for this medication is 0.1 to 0.4 mg qd. This dosage is over 10 times too large.

Body System: Endocrine

1.   **Which condition would most likely be treated with dexamethasone (Decadron)?**

      A.   High blood glucose from Type II diabetes
      B.   A bladder infection from a gram-negative organism
      C.   Increased intracranial pressure from head trauma
      D.   Peptic ulcers secondary to aspirin administration

2   **Identify a normal adult dose of dexamethasone (Decadron)?**

      A.   150 mg PO q 4 hours
      B.   4 mg IV q 6 hours
      C.   0.125 mg IM, q 12 hours
      D.   1 gram IVPB q 6 hours

3.   **What is a common side effect for a client receiving dexamethasone (Decadron)?**

      A.   Low blood sugar and potassium overload
      B.   Sedation and respiratory depression
      C.   Susceptibility to infection
      D.   Bone marrow suppression and renal failure

1.
Answer: C
Rationale:　　　This medication is a steroid that decreases inflammation of the brain tissues and intracranial pressure.

Body System: Endocrine

2.
Answer: B
Rationale:　　　After an initial loading dose of up to 24 mg IV, the normal dosage range is 4-6 mg IV q 6 hours.

Body System: Endocrine

3.
Answer: C
Rationale:　　　Steroid medications suppress the immune system and make the client more susceptible to infections. They also may develop moon face or buffalo hump.

Body System: Endocrine

1.   A client is admitted to the hospital with burns over 20% of the
        body, and the physician orders silver sulfadiazine (Silvadine).
        How should the nurse administer this medication?

        A.   Must be taken with a full glass of water to prevent GI
                irritation
        B.   Give IV push slowly 1 mL per minute
        C.   Should be applied liberally to the burned skin areas
        D.   Give deep IM using the Z-track method

2.   The nurse should question an order for mannitol (Osmitrol) if it
        appears on which client's chart?

        A.   An 88-year-old client in congestive heart failure
        B.   A 44-year-old client with acute glaucoma
        C.   A 22-year-old client with increased intracranial pressure
        D.   An 11-year-old client with acute renal failure

3.   A nurse has just given a client heparin, 50,000 units IV, realizes
        the error and notifies the client's physician. Which nursing inter-
        vention should the nurse probably do next?

        A.   Monitor the client for side effects
        B.   Consult with another nurse about the highest priority
                nursing diagnosis for the client's care plan
        C.   Chart the medication as given and start AM care
        D.   Administer protamine sulfate IV

1.
Answer: C
Rationale: This is a topical antimicrobial cream that is spread over the burned areas of the body.

Body System: Skin

2.
Answer: A
Rationale: This medication pulls fluid into the vascular system from the tissues and would make CHF worse.

Body System: Neurology

3.
Answer: D
Rationale: This dosage is 10 times larger than the normal dose for heparin; protamine sulfate is the correct antidote.

Body System: Cardiovascular

1.   **Which is a side effect often associated with chloramphenicol (Chloromycetin)?**

    A.   Elevated blood sugar
    B.   Sodium retention
    C.   Aplastic anemia
    D.   Cushing's Syndrome

2.   **Which intervention should be included in a teaching plan for a client who is receiving chemotherapeutic agents for cancer?**

    A.   Drink 2,000 to 3,000 mL of fluid per day
    B.   Stay in the direct sunlight as much as possible to increase the production of natural vitamin D
    C.   Eat only when they feel like it to prevent nausea
    D.   Take large doses of acetaminophen (Tylenol) for the pain and discomfort of the disease

3.   **By which route should the nurse give bisacodyl (Dulcolax) to client?**

    A.   IV or IM
    B.   Rectal suppository or IV
    C.   PO or IM
    D.   PO or rectal suppository

1.
Answer: C
Rationale: This is a common and serious side effect of this antibiotic medication.

Body System: Antibiotics

2.
Answer: A
Rationale: Extra fluid is required to rid the body of the medications and prevent damage to the kidneys.

Body System: Chemotherapy

3.
Answer: D
Rationale: This medication comes in a tablet and a rectal suppository only.

Body System: Gastrointestinal

1.   A client who is receiving bisacodyl (Dulcolax) would most likely
        have which condition?

        A.   Acute asthma attacks
        B.   Angina pectoris
        C.   Constipation
        D.   Aplastic anemia

2.   Which medication has an antagonistic effect to bisacodyl
        (Dulcolax)?

        A.   Diphenoxylate (Lomotil)
        B.   Isoniazid (INH)
        C.   Digoxin (Lanoxin)
        D.   Cefaclor (Ceclor)

3.   Which condition requires a client to receive diltiazem (Cardizem)?

        A.   Acute asthma attack
        B.   Angina pectoris
        C.   Constipation
        D.   Aplastic anemia

1.
Answer: C
Rationale: This is a stimulant laxative that is used to treat constipation.

Body System: Gastrointestinal

2.
Answer: A
Rationale: This medication decreases intestinal motility to control diarrhea and will counteract the effects of Dulcolax.

Body System: Gastrointestinal

3.
Answer: B
Rationale: This calcium channel blocker reduces the work load of the heart, reducing oxygen demands and chest pain.

Body System: Cardiovascular

1.   **What are the common side effects that a client receiving diltiazem (Cardizem) may experience?**

        A.   Renal failure, deafness and vision loss
        B.   Low blood pressure, AV block and weakness
        C.   Respiratory depression and muscle paralysis
        D.   Moon face and hyperglycemia

2.   **For which condition would a client be receiving amphetamine (Dexedrine) three times a day?**

        A.   Angina pectoris
        B.   Hyperthyroidism
        C.   Narcolepsy
        D.   Encephalitis

3.   **What side effects would a client most likely experience from amphetamine (Dexedrine)?**

        A.   Respiratory depression and bradycardia
        B.   Postural hypotension and diarrhea
        C.   Drowsiness and loss of muscle coordination
        D.   Dry mouth and weight loss

1.
Answer: B
Rationale: Calcium channel blockers tend to dilate blood vessels and affect the conduction system of the heart.

Body System: Cardiovascular

2.
Answer: C
Rationale: These are very powerful central nervous system stimulants and also are very addictive. Their use is limited to very few diseases including narcolepsy and ADHD.

Body System: Neurology

3.
Answer: D
Rationale: This medication suppresses appetite and has some anticholinergic effects including dry mouth, tachycardia and constipation.

Body System: Neurology

1.   **Which medication would likely produce damage or impairment to the host defense mechanisms?**

    A.   Dextromethorphan (DM)
    B.   Lactulose
    C.   Aminocaproic acid (Amicar)
    D.   Methylprednisolone (Solu-Medrol)

2   **A nursing student is in the Emergency Department observing a clinical experience when an RN hurries out of treatment room 3 and asks the student to run to the pharmacy and get an ampule of aminocaproic acid (Amicar) immediately. The student, on the way to the pharmacy, surmises that the client needs Aminocaproic acid (Amicar) for which reason?**

    A.   An acute asthma attack
    B.   An anaphylactic reaction
    C.   An overdose of streptokinase
    D.   Cardiogenic shock

3.   **Identify the condition a client has who is receiving lactulose along with an antibiotic.**

    A.   Upper respiratory infection and constipation
    B.   Hepatic coma
    C.   Acute alcohol intoxication
    D.   Hypothyroidism

1.
Answer: D
Rationale: Steroid medications suppress the immune system and make the client more susceptible to infections.

Body System: General

2.
Answer: C
Rationale: This medication is used as an antidote for streptokinase and other types of IV anticoagulants.

Body System: Cardiovascular

3.
Answer: B
Rationale: The antibiotic kills the bacteria in the intestines preventing protein digestion and absorption while the lactulose binds with the protein, and removes it through its cathartic action.

Body System: General

1. **What is the classification of cephradine (Velosef)?**

    A.   Antihypertensive
    B.   Antihyperglycemic
    C.   Antibiotic
    D.   Antineoplastic

2. **A 72-year-old client with cancer is to receive nutritional feeding at 75 mL per hour per peg tube. What is the best rationale for this client to receive nutritional feeding?**

    A.   Medication is effective for the client's cancer
    B.   Nutritional feeding will supply one calorie per mL
    C.   Nutritional feeding will maintain normal nutrition
    D.   This is given to prolong life

3. **A nurse is preparing to give a client a dose of propranolol (Inderal). The client says to the nurse "This pill is yellow, the one I usually take is green." What is the best response of the nurse to the client's comment?**

    A.   Encourage the client to take the pill explaining that different medication companies make the same pills in different colors
    B.   Encourage the client to take the pill explaining that it is very important to never stop taking the medication suddenly
    C.   Consult with another nurse who is in the room about whether or not the client should take the medication
    D.   Hold the medication and recheck the dosage with the physician's order

1.
Answer: C
Rationale: This is a synthetic cephalosporin, broad spectrum antibiotic.

Body System: General

2.
Answer: B
Rationale: Often cancer clients are unable to eat enough to maintain normal nutrition; high calorie supplements are sometimes used to provide calories and proteins.

Body System: General

3.
Answer: D
Rationale: Clients often know what medications they are taking. Any questions they raise about the medication should be evaluated before administering it.

Body System: General

1.   As part of the treatment regimen for a client's peptic ulcer, the physician orders cimetidine (Tagamet). What is the correct dosage for this medication?

    A.   300 mg PO four times a day
    B.   50 mg PO bid with meals
    C.   10 mg IM every two hours
    D.   500 mg PO each morning

2.   Which statement by the client will indicate to the nurse that teaching about ranitidine (Zantac) has been effective?

    A.   "I need to always take the medication on an empty stomach."
    B.   "Smoking will decrease the effectiveness of the medication."
    C.   "I need to always take the medication with food or milk."
    D.   "When I feel better, I can stop taking the medication."

3.   A client with a peptic ulcer does not respond well to cimetidine (Tagamet). The physician changes the medication to ranitidine (Zantac). How does ranitidine differ from cimetidine?

    A.   It is less potent than Tagamet and requires a larger dose
    B.   Ranitidine works on a different mechanism than Tagamet
    C.   It is more potent than Tagamet and requires a smaller dose
    D.   There is no difference between the medications

1.
Answer: A
Rationale: The dosage range for an adult is 300 mg ac and hs.

Body System: Gastrointestinal

2.
Answer: B
Rationale: Smoking stimulates the production of gastric secretions and will counteract the effect of the medication.

Body System: Gastrointestinal

3.
Answer: C
Rationale: It is stronger and requires less to produce similar results.

Body System: Gastrointestinal

1. **The physician orders sucralfate (Carafate) for a client. It is most likely that the client has which problem?**

   A. Diarrhea
   B. Ileitis
   C. Esophagitis
   D. Anorexia

2. **What is true about an order for 1 gram of sucralfate (Carafate) PO, four times a day for a client who has a peptic ulcer?**

   A. The dose is correct for the condition
   B. The dose is much too large and may be lethal
   C. The dose is too small to be effective
   D. The physician made a mistake when ordering the medication

3. **What important factor should the nurse keep in mind when administering sucralfate (Carafate) to a client?**

   A. It works best if it is taken with food
   B. It works best if taken on an empty stomach
   C. The B/P and pulse must be taken before the medication can be given
   D. Diarrhea is the most common side effect

1.
Answer: C
Rationale: This medication is a standard treatment for irritations of the upper GI tract including esophagitis, gastritis and peptic ulcers.

Body System: Gastrointestinal

2.
Answer: A
Rationale: This is the correct dosage for this medication.

Body System: Gastrointestinal

3.
Answer: B
Rationale: It should be given on an empty stomach one-half to one hour before meals.

Body System: Gastrointestinal

1.   **What is the classification of psyllium (Metamucil)?**

   A.   Surfactant laxative
   B.   Stimulant cathartic
   C.   Bulk-forming laxative
   D.   Anti-anginal agent

2.   **What is the most likely reason that a client with angina pectoris would be taking psyllium (Metamucil)?**

   A.   Relieve chest pain
   B.   Prevent from having diarrhea
   C.   Help stay on bed rest
   D.   Prevent straining from constipation

3.   **For which condition is psyllium (Metamucil) sometimes prescribed?**

   A.   Peptic ulcer disease
   B.   Diverticulitis
   C.   Gastroenteritis
   D.   Achalasia

1.
Answer: C
Rationale: This medication expands in the GI tract when water is drawn into it from the tissues. Promotes normal bowel movements.

Body System: Gastrointestinal

2.
Answer: D
Rationale: Straining to have a BM in clients with cardiac disease can increase chest pain or cause dysrhythmias.

Body System: Gastrointestinal

3.
Answer: B
Rationale: This medication keeps the stool soft and prevents irritation of the intestinal linings.

Body System: Gastrointestinal

1. **Which is an important factor that the nurse should remember in administering psyllium (Metamucil) to a client?**

   A. The medication should be mixed 60 minutes ahead of time
   B. The medication should be taken with food
   C. When mixed in juice, medication should be followed by a glass of water
   D. Take the client's B/P and pulse before administering

2. **A 32-year-old accountant is diagnosed with inflammatory bowel syndrome (Crohn's Disease). Which medication is most likely to be included in the treatment regimen?**

   A. Psyllium (Metamucil)
   B. Diphenoxylate (Lomotil)
   C. Dimenhydrinate (Dramamine)
   D. Lactulose (Chronulac)

3. **A physician orders prochlorperazine (Compazine) 50 mg IV every four hours as needed for nausea and vomiting for a 74-year-old client with a diagnosis of flu. What is the best response by the nurse to this order?**

   A. Give the medication as soon as possible to prevent further dehydration from fluid loss during vomiting
   B. Don't give the medication and notify the physician that Compazine is not effective for this type of nausea
   C. Give the medication as ordered but monitor the client for side effects
   D. Don't give the medication and notify the physician that the dose is too large

1.
Answer: C
Rationale: Because this medication relies upon the absorption of water for its effects, additional fluid is required.

Body System: Gastrointestinal

2.
Answer: B
Rationale: This condition is marked by excessive diarrhea — this medication controls that problem.

Body System: Gastrointestinal

3.
Answer: D
Rationale: Normal dosage range for an adult is 5-10 mg IV.

Body System: Gastrointestinal

1. **What common side effects should be monitored while a client is receiving prochlorperazine (Compazine)?**

   A. Diarrhea, urinary retention and tachycardia
   B. Drowsiness, respiratory depression and hypotension
   C. Alopecia, bleeding and bone marrow suppression
   D. Bradycardia, renal failure and anxiety

2. **A 43-year-old business person takes dimenhydrinate (Dramamine) for motion sickness when flying. What is an important factor to remember in relation to this medication?**

   A. It works best if started 2 days prior to activity (flying)
   B. It should be taken with food but not much fluid
   C. It should be taken 30 to 60 minutes before flying
   D. It should be followed by 60 mL of water

3. **What is the normal dosage range for dimenhydrinate (Dramamine)?**

   A. 10 to 20 mg PO q 4 - 6 hrs PRN
   B. 50 to 100 mg PO q 4 - 6 hrs PRN
   C. 150 to 200 mg PO q 4 - 6 hrs PRN
   D. 250 to 500 mg PO q 4 - 6 hrs PRN

1.
Answer: B
Rationale: This medication tends to suppress the central nervous
                     system and lowers blood pressure.

Body System: Gastrointestinal

2.
Answer: C
Rationale: It is most effective if taken before flying so that it can
                     absorb into the system.

Body System: Gastrointestinal

3.
Answer: B
Rationale: This is the normal range — may also be given IM or IV.

Body System: Gastrointestinal

1.   **What disease would a client who is admitted with an order for lactulose (Chronulac) most likely have?**

      A.   Diabetes mellitus
      B.   Chronic diarrhea
      C.   Wilson's disease
      D.   Hepatic encephalopathy

2.   **Identify the classification of lactulose (Chronulac).**

      A.   Antacid
      B.   GI stimulant
      C.   Disaccharide cathartic
      D.   Monosaccharide cathartic

3.   **How does lactulose (Chronulac) exert its effect?**

      A.   Stimulates the pancreas to increase the production of insulin
      B.   Slows the propulsive movements in the intestines
      C.   Stimulates the production of mucus in the small and large intestinal linings
      D.   Pulls water into the intestinal lumen

1.
Answer: D
Rationale: This medication is used in conjunction with antibiotics to decrease the ammonia level in the blood.

Body System: Gastrointestinal

2.
Answer: C
Rationale: It is used to prevent protein breakdown in the digestive system.

Body System: Gastrointestinal

3.
Answer: D
Rationale: These medications soften the stool by pulling water into the fecal material.

Body System: Gastrointestinal

1.   **Which medication is a powerful agent that promotes cleansing of the bowel?**

       A.   Laxative
       B.   Cathartic
       C.   An antidiarrheal
       D.   Antiemetic

2.   **What is the normal dose range for lactulose (Chronulac) by mouth?**

       A.   10 - 50 mg bid
       B.   15 - 30 mL qd
       C.   100 - 300 mcg qid
       D.   1 - 2 grams qod

3.   **What types of clients usually take docusate (Surfak)?**

       A.   Clients in whom straining to stool is potentially harmful
       B.   Clients who require cleansing of the bowel before endoscopic procedures
       C.   Clients with a fecal impaction
       D.   Clients with inflammatory bowel disease

1.
Answer: B
Rationale: These medications irritate the bowel and cause increased peristalsis.

Body System: Gastrointestinal

2.
Answer: B
Rationale: This is the normal range — medication can only be given by mouth.

Body System: Gastrointestinal

3.
Answer: A
Rationale: This is a mild laxative that softens stool in clients in whom constipation may be a problem.

Body System: Gastrointestinal

1.   **Which action interferes most with the effects of bisacodyl (Dulco-lax) tablets?**

        A.   Swallowing the tablets without chewing
        B.   Avoid taking the medications with milk or antacids
        C.   Take the medication with H_2 inhibitors
        D.   Take the medication with meals

2.   **Which medication normally produces the fastest results when taken by mouth?**

        A.   Psyllium (Metamucil)
        B.   Docusate (Surfak)
        C.   Bisacodyl (Dulcolax)
        D.   Lactulose (Chronulac)

3.   **What class of medications decreases the effectiveness of laxatives and cathartics?**

        A.   Anticholinergics
        B.   Cholinergics
        C.   CNS stimulants
        D.   Antibiotics

1.
Answer: C
Rationale: The H_2 inhibitors decrease peristalsis and reduce the effectiveness of the medication.

Body System: Gastrointestinal

2.
Answer: C
Rationale: This medication is the fastest acting of the PO laxatives-effective in a few hours.

Body System: Gastrointestinal

3.
Answer: A
Rationale: These medications slow the peristalsis of the GI tract.

Body System: Gastrointestinal

1.   **What is the action of docusate (Surfak)?**

      A.   Strong laxative
      B.   Antibiotic
      C.   Stool softener
      D.   Vaccine

2.   **An antineoplastic medication regimen is considered successful when what percentage of the cancer cells are killed?**

      A.   90%
      B.   95%
      C.   99%
      D.   100%

3.   **Why are combinations of antineoplastic medications commonly used in the treatment of cancer?**

      A.   Prevents or delays the development of resistance
      B.   Increases the length of treatment
      C.   Increases the quantity of each medication used
      D.   Prevents serious side effects

1.
Answer: C
Rationale: Acts to permit water and fatty substances to be well mixed
with fecal material.

Body System: Gastrointestinal

2.
Answer: D
Rationale: All the cancer cells must be killed or they are likely to
regrow.

Body System: Chemotherapy

3.
Answer: A
Rationale: Different medications work on different parts of the growth
cycle of tumor cells and helps prevent resistant cells from
developing.

Body System: Chemotherapy

1. **What is the normal pattern for the administration of antineoplastic medications?**

    A.   Low doses given continually over a long period of time
    B.   Massive doses given only once
    C.   Relatively high doses on a cyclic schedule
    D.   IV medications alternating with PO medications

2. **What is the primary reason for the cyclic pattern of administration with antineoplastic medications?**

    A.   Decreases the long term cost to the client
    B.   Increases the cell kill gradually
    C.   Produces less immunosuppression
    D.   Does not allow the cancer cells to reproduce

3. **Which diet is appropriate for a client receiving vincristine (Oncovin)?**

    A.   Strained fruit juices and refined breads
    B.   Cottage cheese and whole milk
    C.   Raw vegetables and whole grain cereals
    D.   Herbs, spices and salt

1.
Answer: C
Rationale: The high doses produce the maximum destruction of cancer cells (the cyclical schedule allows the bone marrow to recover between administrations).

Body System: Chemotherapy

2.
Answer: C
Rationale: Allows the bone marrow and immune systems to recover between cycles.

Body System: Chemotherapy

3.
Answer: C
Rationale: This medication causes constipation and this diet increases fiber.

Body System: Chemotherapy

1.   **What is the mode of action of surfactant laxatives?**

        A.   Draws extra water into the small intestine
        B.   Prevents the absorption of the digested food
        C.   Decreases the surface tension of the stool
        D.   Increases the bulk in the stool

2.   **For which condition would a client most likely be receiving metoclopramide (Reglan)?**

        A.   Cancer of the liver
        B.   Gastroesophageal reflux
        C.   Crohn's disease
        D.   Ulcerative colitis

3.   **What is the normal adult dosage range for metoclopramide (Reglan)?**

        A.   2 - 5 mg PO ac and hs
        B.   10 - 15 mg PO ac and hs
        C.   50 - 75 mg IM tid
        D.   150 - 300 mg PO pc and hs

1.
Answer: C
Rationale: These laxatives act like soap and break down the molecular adhesion of water molecules allowing the stools to absorb more water.

Body System: Gastrointestinal

2.
Answer: B
Rationale: Medication is used for conditions of the upper GI tract including nausea, vomiting, and delayed gastric emptying.

Body System: Gastrointestinal

3.
Answer: B
Rationale: This is the correct dosage range for this medication — may also be given IV.

Body System: Gastrointestinal

1. **What is an important nursing implication to consider when giving a client metoclopramide (Reglan)?**

   A.   Increase fluid intake to 3,000 to 5,000 mL per day
   B.   Take the medication with meals or milk
   C.   Monitor pulse and B/P
   D.   Avoid giving the medication with anticholinergics

2. **How will a client with chest pain know that the nitroglycerin SL being taken is effective?**

   A.   A burning or tingling sensation when placed under the tongue
   B.   Chest pain is relieved
   C.   Blood pressure drops after five minutes
   D.   Heart rate decreases after two minutes

3. **Which is an important factor for a client to remember when taking sublingual nitroglycerin?**

   A.   Drink 60 mL of water with the medication to prevent stomach ulcers
   B.   Take the medication with food
   C.   Sit or lie down when taking the medication
   D.   Call the physician whenever he or she has to take more than one

1.
Answer: D
Rationale: Anticholinergic medications decrease the action and
effectiveness of this medication.

Body System: Gastrointestinal

2.
Answer: B
Rationale: The purpose of taking this medication is to relieve the chest
pain — the only measure of effectiveness.

Body System: Cardiovascular

3.
Answer: C
Rationale: Common side effect is postural hypotension from the
vasodilating effects, and can lead to dizziness and syncope.

Body System: Cardiovascular

1. **Which medication is effective in treating a client with a ventricular dysrhythmia secondary to digoxin toxicity?**

    A.   Lidocaine HCI
    B.   Quinidine (Quinidex)
    C.   Phenytoin (Dilantin)
    D.   Verapamil (Calan)

2. **Which statement voiced by the client will indicate that the nurse's teaching concerning verapamil (Calan) has been successful?**

    A.   "I can stop taking this medication when I begin to feel like my old self."
    B.   "If I begin to feel dizzy, weak or have swelling in my ankles, I need to notify my physician."
    C.   "If I miss a dose, I need to double up on the next dose."
    D.   "I must take this medication with meals so that it doesn't upset my stomach."

3. **Which medication is effective in treating a client with a second degree AV heart block?**

    A.   Lidocaine
    B.   Epinephrine
    C.   Atropine
    D.   Quinidine

1.
Answer: C
Rationale: This medication has effects similar to lidocaine but is effective in the presence of elevated lanoxin levels.

Body System: Cardiovascular

2.
Answer: B
Rationale: Common side effects of this medication are hypotension, bradycardia and peripheral edema.

Body System: Cardiovascular

3.
Answer: C
Rationale: Atropine sulfate, 0.5 to 1.0 mg IV is used to treat most slow heart rate conditions including AV blocks and bradycardia.

Body System: Cardiovascular

1. **What medication would likely be used for a client who goes into ventricular asystole?**

   A.   Lanoxin 0.5 mg IV push
   B.   Epinephrine 1 amp IV push
   C.   NTG gr 1/150 sl stat
   D.   Diltiazem 90 mg PO

2. **A Pronestyl drip (mixed 2 grams of Pronestyl in 500 mL of D₅W) is started on a client. It is to run at 4 mg per minute. At what rate should the volumetric pump be set?**

   A.   33 mL/hr
   B.   7.5 mL/hr
   C.   60 mL/hr
   D.   30 mL/hr

3. **A client is started on a heparin drip that is mixed 20,000 units in 500 mL of D₅W. It is to run at 1600 units per hour. At what rate should the volumetric pump be set to deliver this dosage of medication?**

   A.   40 mL/hr
   B.   60 mL/hr
   C.   10 mL/hr
   D.   16 mL/hr

1.
Answer: B
Rationale: Epinephrine is a very powerful cardiac stimulant and will
                   produce cardiac contractions in a cardiac arrest situation.

<u>Body System: Cardiovascular</u>

2.
Answer: C
Rationale: Math: concentration = $\frac{2000}{500}$ = 4 mg/mL

                   mg/hr = 4 mg/min X 60 min = 240 mg/hr

                   mL/hr = $\frac{240}{4}$ = 60 mL/hr

<u>Body System: Cardiovascular</u>

3.
Answer: A
Rationale: Math: Concentration = $\frac{20,000}{500}$ = 40 units/mL

                   mL/hr = $\frac{1,600}{40}$ = 40 mL/hr

<u>Body System: Cardiovascular</u>

1.   **Which medication is most appropriate to use in the treatment of a client who has just developed paroxysmal atrial tachycardia?**

   A.   Lidocaine 75 mg IV push
   B.   Lanoxin 0.25 mg IV push
   C.   Atropine Sulfate 1 mg IV push
   D.   Verapamil 5 mg IV push

2.   **Which medications are used for supraventricular tachydysrythmias?**

   A.   Atropine and bretylium (Bretylol)
   B.   Quinidine (Quinaglute) and lidocaine
   C.   Propranolol (Inderal) and verapamil (Calan)
   D.   Epinephrine and dopamine (Intropin)

3.   **Which medication is good to use for atrioventricular blocks?**

   A.   Lidocaine and bretylium (Bretylol)
   B.   Propranolol (Inderal) and verapamil (Calan)
   C.   Quinidine (Quinaglute) and dopamine (Intropin)
   D.   Atropine and epinephrine (Adrenalin)

1.
Answer: D
Rationale: This calcium channel blocker has been very successful in treating dysrhythmia.

Body System: Cardiovascular

2.
Answer: C
Rationale: These two medications are generally effective in controlling dysrhythmias.

Body System: Cardiovascular

3.
Answer: D
Rationale: These are effective in increasing the rate in A-V blocks.

Body System: Cardiovascular

1. How many teaspoons of aluminum hydroxide (Maalox) will be administered to give 0.5 ounces?

   A.   1 tsp
   B.   2 tsp
   C.   3 tsp
   D.   4 tsp

2. The nurse is to give phenobarbital gr 1/2 in liquid form. The label on the bottle states that there are 20 mg/5 cc of the medication. How many cc's should the nurse administer?

   A.   2.5 cc
   B.   5 cc
   C.   7.5 cc
   D.   10 cc

3. The nurse is to give penicillin 350,000 u. The vial contains 100,000 u per 1.6 cc. The nurse will administer how many cc?

   A.   4.6 cc
   B.   4.5 cc
   C.   6 cc
   D.   5.6 cc

1.
Answer: C
Rationale: One teaspoon is equal to 5 cc. 1 ounce = 30 cc. 1/2 ounce
= 15 cc. 15 cc = 3 teaspoons.

Body System: Gastrointestinal

2.
Answer: C
Rationale: 2. 60 mg = 1 grain (gr) gr1/2 = 30 mg. Using the formula
Desired x solution, the problem is set up:
Have

$\frac{30\ mg}{20\ mg}$ x 5 cc = 1.5 x 5 = 7.5 cc

Body System: Neurology

3.
Answer: D
Rationale: Using Desired   x solution, the problem is set up:
Have

$\frac{350,000}{100,000}$ x 1.6 cc = 3.5 x 1.6 = 5.6 cc

Body System: Antibiotics

1.   A nurse is to give cephalexin (Keflex) 0.75 gm. The tablets are labeled in mgs. To give the correct dose, how many milligrams should be given?

      A.   .75
      B.   7.5
      C.   75
      D.   750

2.   The physician's orders read: "Digoxin (Lanoxin) 0.25 mg." Scored tablets are 0.125 mg each. How many tablets should the nurse administer?

      A.   1/4
      B.   1/2
      C.   1 1/2
      D.   2

3.   The physician has ordered a medication qid. The nurse will best schedule the medication administration at which of the following times?

      A.   8 am, 4 pm, 12 midnight
      B.   8 am, 8 pm
      C.   8 am, 2 pm, 8 pm, 2 am
      D.   8 am, 12 noon, 5 pm, 9 pm

1.
Answer: D
Rationale: Convert .75 gm to mgs   1000 mg = 1 gm
                        .75 x 1000 = 750 mg

Body System: Antibiotics

2.
Answer: D
Rationale: Use formula <u>Desired</u>
                              Have

                   Set up problem <u>.25 mg</u>
                                   .125 mg = 2 tablets

Body System: Cardiovascular

3.
Answer: D
Rationale: QID means four times a day. This is best done by
                   scheduling the medications at equal intervals apart; 8 am, 12
                   noon, 5 pm, 9 pm.

Body System: General

1.   **What is the action of a Beta 2 antagonist?**

   A.   Blocks Beta 2 receptors
   B.   Has no effect on Beta 2
   C.   Stimulates Beta 2 receptors
   D.   Stops a Beta 2 response from occurring

2.   **What is the purpose of interferon?**

   A.   Induces uninfected cells to produce alterations that protect
           those cells from viral multiplication
   B.   Ingests foreign particulate matter and damaged host tissues
   C.   Forms a thin layer of epithelial cells over a wound and
           deposits fibrin in the wound
   D.   Stimulates the sympathetic adrenal medullary mechanisms
           during the stress response

3.   **The nurse adds medications to an IV bottle and notes that the
        solution   becomes cloudy. What are the proper actions and
        correct rationale?**

   A.   Do not hang the bottle since clouding indicates a reaction
           has taken place, and the solution should not be administered
   B.   Hang the bottle; there is no danger if particles are not
           visible
   C.   Hang the bottle, but put an inline filter between the bottle
           and the client; any particle will be stopped
   D.   Do not hang the bottle; call the physician and do as
           instructed

1.
Answer: C
Rationale: Antagonist refers to stimulation of receptors. Beta antagonists block beta receptors and prevent the beta stimulation from occurring.

Body System: Cardiovascular

2.
Answer: A
Rationale: Interferon is thought to prevent the replication of viruses. It does not ingest foreign material. Fibrinogen forms fibrin over the wound. Interferon has no effect on the adrenal medulla.

Body System: Endocrine

3.
Answer: A
Rationale: Any change in the solution color indicates precipitation has occurred. The solution cannot be hung as the precipitated solution may lead to emboli introduction into the blood stream. The physician will not need to be notified as the client has not been harmed, and the nurse can correct the situation by hanging one IV medication at a time.

Body System: General

1.   **Why should the nurse not want the drip chamber to become full?**

      A.   Air would be allowed to enter
      B.   The solution would back up
      C.   You could not count the drops
      D.   It is okay for tube chamber to be full

2.   **What should the nurse do before spiking and hanging the bottle?**

      A.   Clamp the tubing
      B.   Clean the spike
      C.   Count the drops
      D.   Unclamp the tubing

3.   **Which is true of a correctly administered intradermal injection?**

      A.   The needle is held at a 30° angle to the skin surface
      B.   The nurse will aspirate for blood prior to giving the injection
      C.   The site must be circled for reading as the skin surface remains flat
      D.   The area should not be massaged after the injection

1.
Answer: C
Rationale: If the drip chamber is too full, the nurse cannot see the drops fall and cannot count the flow rate. Air will not enter if the drip chamber is full. The solution will not back up, even if the drip chamber is full.

Body System: General

2.
Answer: A
Rationale: The tubing should be clamped to prevent fluid from proceeding down the IV tubing interspersed with air. The spike is considered sterile when unwrapped and would not need cleaning. The nurse cannot count the drops until the IV is running. Tubing comes unclamped when taken out of the box it comes in.

Body System: General

3.
Answer: D
Rationale: A correctly administered injection is given at a 20° angle. Aspiration is not necessary as no blood vessels are present in the intradermal tissue. The production of a wheal indicates that the medication is in the intradermal space rather than the subcutaneous tissue.

Body System: General

1. **What is the preferred site of administration for an IM injection in an adult?**

   A.   Vastus lateralis muscle
   B.   Deltoid muscle
   C.   Gluteus medius muscle
   D.   Rectus femoris muscle

2. **To administer ear drops to an adult, how should the nurse pull the pinna (outer side of the ear)?**

   A.   Down and forward
   B.   Back and down
   C.   Up and forward
   D.   Up and back

3. **A client is to receive eye drops in the left eye. What is the correct abbreviation for left eye?**

   A.   OD
   B.   OL
   C.   OS
   D.   OU

1.
Answer: C
Rationale: Gluteus medius muscle is well developed in the adult. The
vastus lateralis and rectus femoris muscles of the legs may
result in greater discomfort later, as these muscles may be
used more frequently than the gluteus medius muscle. There
is generally greater muscle mass at the gluteus medius site
than at the deltoid site in the adult.

Body System: General

2.
Answer: D
Rationale: Pulling the pinna of the ear up and back will straighten the
ear canal. Down and forward or up and forward will not
straighten the canal. Back and down straightens the canal of
an infant.

Body System: Ear/topical

3.
Answer: C
Rationale: The abbreviation OS means left eye, the abbreviation OD
means right eye. OU refers to both eyes. OL is not a usual
abbreviation referring to the eye.

Body System: Eye/topical

1. The nurse is preparing 9 a.m. medications at 9:30 a.m., and is not familiar with one of the medications. Given this situation, the nurse should:

    A. Give all but the unfamiliar one, look it up, and give it at the next scheduled time
    B. Give all the medications, and then immediately look up the side effects of the unfamiliar one
    C. Don't give any of the medications since it's 30 minutes past time to give them
    D. Look up the unfamiliar medication, then proceed to give all the medications

2. After inserting the needle for an intramuscular injection, which nursing action should be next?

    A. Inject the medication
    B. Pull back on the plunger
    C. Pull the needle back 1/8 inch
    D. Squeeze the tissue more firmly

3. The intravenous order reads: "1000 cc D_5 W over 10 hr." What would the nurse determine to be gtts/min with a drip set (15 gtts/cc)?

    A. 15
    B. 25
    C. 34
    D. 100

1.
Answer: D
Rationale: The nurse should never give medications with which he or
she is not familiar, even if it is late giving medications.
Medications are considered to be administered on time if
given within one half hour of the scheduled time. Even if
medications are given late, they should still be given, but
the actual time given should be charted.

Body System: General

2.
Answer: B
Rationale: The nurse will pull back on the plunger to check for
aspiration of blood from a blood vessel. This is necessary
to prevent the possibility of injecting the medication into the
blood stream. Once the needle is inserted, it should not be
pulled back. Tissue should not be squeezed at the time of an
intramuscular injection.

Body System: General

3.
Answer: B
Rationale: An Abbott macrodrip set has 15 drops/cc of fluid. One liter
equals 1000 cc. 1000 cc given over 10 hours equals 100
cc/hour.

Using the formula $\dfrac{Volume}{Time\ in\ minutes}$ x drip factor

set up the problem $\dfrac{1000\ cc}{600\ minutes}$ x 15 = 25 gtts/min

Body System: General

1. The physician's order reads, "Give morphine sulfate gr 1/6 IM every 4 hours PRN for pain." The medication is available in 10 mg/mL ampules. When the client requests pain medication, the nurse administers gr 1/6. How many mgs will the nurse administer?

    A.   1.25 mg
    B.   0.75 mg
    C.   1.0 mg
    D.   .05 mg

2. A client has meperidine (Demerol) 75 mg ordered. The meperidine (Demerol) supply on the unit is Demerol 50 mg = 1 mL. How many mLs should the nurse administer?

    A.   0.2
    B.   0.4
    C.   0.7
    D.   1.5

3. At what rate does a microdrip intravenous set deliver fluid?

    A.   60 gtts/min
    B.   15 gtts/mL
    C.   60 gtt/mL
    D.   Varies with manufacturer

1.
Answer: C
Rationale: 60 mg = 1 grain   1/6 grain = 1.0 mg

Body System: Analgesic

2.
Answer: D
Rationale: Using the formula <u>Desired</u> x solution
                          Have

$$\frac{75 \text{ mg}}{50 \text{ mg}} \times 1 = 1.5 \text{ mL}$$

Body System: Analgesic

3.
Answer: C
Rationale: Microdrips always deliver fluid at 60 drops per milliliter.
Macrodrips deliver at 15 gtts/mL.

Body System: General

1.   **Why is a paracervical block administered to the client to allay pain?**

   A.   Cervical dilatation
   B.   Pain of delivery
   C.   Pain during episiotomy incision
   D.   Pain during episiotomy suturing

2.   **Which route is best to deliver vitamin K to a newborn?**

   A.   Subcutaneously
   B.   Intramuscularly
   C.   Orally
   D.   Rectally

3.   **Which medication is associated with these side effects: drop in BP, perspiration, N & V, and facial flushing?**

   A.   Meperidine (Demerol)
   B.   Promethazine (Phenergan)
   C.   Scopolamine
   D.   Morphine sulfate

1.
Answer: A
Rationale: Local anesthetic injected around the cervix numbs the cervical area relieving only the pain caused by cervical dilatation.

Body System: General

2.
Answer: B
Rationale: Vitamin K is best absorbed from muscle tissue due to its vascularity.

Body System: General

3.
Answer: A
Rationale: These are common side effects of Demerol.

Body System: General

1. **Why is simethicone (Mylicon) frequently given postoperatively?**

   A. Increases peristalsis
   B. Prevents gas distention
   C. Prevents nausea and vomiting
   D. Increases respirations

2. **A client is hospitalized for severe preeclampsia and is started on magnesium sulfate (MgSO₄). Prior to administering a second dose of the medication, the nurse finds the client's patellar tendon flex is +1, respirations are 16 per min., and urine output is 120 mL in the last 4 hours. What is the nurse's priority action as a result of these findings?**

   A. Give $MgSO_4$ as ordered
   B. Give one-half of the $MgSO_4$
   C. Hold the $MgSO_4$ and consult the physician
   D. Give calcium gluconate immediately

3. **Which of the following is the medication of choice to control postpartum hemorrhage?**

   A. Ergotrate gr 1/320 (IV) push
   B. Methergine 0.2 mg (IM) q 4 h
   C. Buccal Pitocin
   D. Pitocin 10 U in 1000 cc D₅W IV over 8 hours

1.
Answer: B
Rationale: Mylicon (Simethicone) acts on the stomach and intestines by dispersing and preventing the formation of mucus surrounding gas pockets.

Body System: Gastrointestinal

2.
Answer: A
Rationale: The findings listed are all within normal limits.

Body System: Neurology/General

3.
Answer: D
Rationale: Delivery of medication over several hours will cause sustained uterine contractions preventing blood loss.

Body System: Obstetric

1. **During which time period is the fetus most likely to be damaged by the pregnant woman's ingestion of medications?**

    A.   First trimester
    B.   Second trimester
    C.   Third trimester
    D.   Entire pregnancy

2. **Which substance is the antidote for magnesium sulfate?**

    A.   Sodium pentothal
    B.   Calcium gluconate
    C.   Calcium chloride
    D.   Calcium carbonate

3. **Select the most common side effects of tetracyclines.**

    A.   Nausea, vomiting, diarrhea, stomatitis
    B.   Deafness, urticaria, pain at injection site
    C.   Slow pulse, pinpoint pupils, diminished reflexes
    D.   Skin rash, constipation, breakthrough bleeding

1.
Answer: A
Rationale: The first trimester is the period of organogenesis-each organ is more vulnerable to teratogenic substances.

Body System: Obstetric

2.
Answer: B
Rationale: Administered over 3 min. IV and repeated every hour until respiratory, urinary and neurologic depression have been alleviated.

Body System: Obstetric

3.
Answer: A
Rationale: These are the most common side effects associated with this medication.

Body System: Antibiotic

1. **Which medication produces amnesia?**

    A.   Loxapine
    B.   Scopolamine
    C.   Atropine
    D.   Benztropine

2. **What is the action of phenobarbital (Luminal)?**

    A.   Causes uterus to contract
    B.   Sedation — anti-convulsant
    C.   Lowers BP
    D.   Enhances Vitamin K synthesis

3. **What is the usual dose of meperidine (Demerol) for a client in labor?**

    A.   15 mg
    B.   150 mg
    C.   50 mg
    D.   200 mg

1.
Answer: B
Rationale: Given in larger doses this medication produces an amnesia effect.

Body System: Neurology

2.
Answer: B
Rationale: Used when seizures are present.

Body System: Neurology

3.
Answer: C
Rationale: This dose is safe for mother and baby. The safe range is 50-100 mg IM or IV in the mid stage of labor.

Body System: Analgesic

1. **What should the nurse check prior to administering ergonovine (Ergotrate Maleate) gr 1/320?**

   A. Blood pressure
   B. Knee jerk reflex
   C. Respirations
   D. Pulse

2. **A client has been on an antidepressant medication for five days. On the sixth day the nurse brings the regular dose of medication and the client says, "I have been taking this pill for a week, and it has not done me any good. Maybe I should get two pills instead of one? Or, maybe, I should stop taking it all together?" What is the best response to this client statement?**

   A. "You are exaggerating. You have only been on the medication for five days."
   B. "You don't have to take the medication if you don't want to. Of course, I will have to notify the physician."
   C. "You feel discouraged because the medication is not working. It may take longer for you to feel the effects of this medication."
   D. "We can talk to the physician about the dosage next time. In the meantime, you must take the medication."

3. **For what reason would Atropine be used for a client who was receiving ECT treatments?**

   A. Diminishes the level of consciousness
   B. Improves oxygenation of tissues
   C. Reduces painful muscle spasms
   D. Reduces secretions and vagal stimulation

Pharmacology Review

1.
Answer: A
Rationale: It is a vasoconstricting medication.

Body System: Obstetric

2.
Answer: C
Rationale: Acknowledges the client's feelings and provides correct information.

Body System: Psychology

3.
Answer: D
Rationale: This is a therapeutic action of Atropine.

Body System: Psychology

1. **A client has ingested half a can of beer after having been on disul-firam (Antabuse) for one week. What is the client likely to experience?**

   A. A feeling of intoxication and euphorias
   B. An intense craving for alcohol
   C. Not much, since he has been on the medication for such a short period of time
   D. Pounding headache, nausea, vomiting and hypotension

2. **What is the primary purpose for placing an opiate-dependent person on methadone (Dolophine)?**

   A. Alter the person's basic dependent personality structure
   B. Assist the person to live a life free of "street drugs"
   C. Prevent complications from opiates
   D. Study the effects of the medication on the personality

3. **In assessing a client who abuses substances, which disadvantage associated with a high intake of amphetamines poses the greatest immediate danger for the drug abuser?**

   A. Psychological dependence on the medication
   B. Paranoid from taking the medication
   C. Depressed and suicidal between doses of the medication
   D. Develops an infection from self-administration of the medication

1.
Answer: D
Rationale: These symptoms occur because acetaldehyde builds up in the body.

Body System: Psychology

2.
Answer: B
Rationale: Methadone minimizes opiate cravings, providing the opportunity for a functional, productive life.

Body System: Psychology

3.
Answer: C
Rationale: Depression and suicidal behavior may occur when the medication blood level is low.

Body System: Psychology

1. Some narcotic addicts enter the hospital voluntarily to withdraw from a medication. It has been observed that occasionally following withdrawal, an addict dies from the first dose of the addicting medication taken afterward. Which of these statements helps to explain this fact?

    A.   To get the desired effect after a period of forced abstinence, addicts need more than the customary dose of medication previously taken
    B.   Medication withdrawal causes temporary impairment in an addict's mental faculties
    C.   Withdrawal reduces the addict's medication tolerance
    D.   The development of an allergic reaction to the addicting medication is very common following withdrawal

2. What may be caused by rapid withdrawal from barbiturates?

    A.   Fatigue and depression
    B.   Excruciating abdominal pain
    C.   Tremors and convulsions
    D.   Hallucinations and panic state

3. Which category of medication (psychoactive agents) is most commonly used in the management of children with attention deficit hyperactive disorder?

    A.   Antidepressants
    B.   Antipsychotics
    C.   Cerebral stimulant
    D.   Sedatives and hypnotics

1.
Answer: C
Rationale: Tolerance decreases during abstinence. Decreased tolerance can lead to coma, shock and respiratory depression.

Body System: Psychology

2.
Answer: C
Rationale: Convulsions and cardiovascular complications are the most dangerous complications of rapid withdrawal.

Body System: Psychology

3.
Answer: C
Rationale: Central nervous stimulants are most often prescribed.

Body System: Psychology

1.   A client glares at the nurse suspiciously when approached with
        medicine. As the nurse extends the medicine cup, the client says,
        "I'm not going to take it. Who ordered it? What's it for?" Which
        nursing action is most therapeutic?

        A.   Explain the general purpose of the medication
        B.   Notify the physician of the client's refusal to take the
                medication
        C.   Simply document in the record that the client refused
                medication
        D.   Tell the client he/she is being non-compliant and further
                treatment may not be ordered.

2.   A client has been placed on amitriptyline (Elavil). What signs
        should the nurse look for when evaluating the effects of amitrip-
        tyline (Elavil)?

        A.   Anorexia, confusion, and coma
        B.   Dehydration, diarrhea, and muscle weakness
        C.   Dry mouth, blurred vision, and constipation
        D.   Polyuria, pulse irregularities, and slurred speech

3.   A client has a history of mood swings from depression to elation.
        The client is currently displaying signs of mania. Which treatment
        will probably be used for the client?

        A.   Antidepressant medications
        B.   Sedative medications
        C.   Lithium carbonate
        D.   ECT (electroconvulsive therapy)

1.
Answer: A
Rationale: Correct information will decrease anxiety.

Body System: Psychology

2.
Answer: D
Rationale: Most common side effects related to the anticholinergic effect.

Body System: Psychology

3.
Answer: C
Rationale: Treatment of choice for manic depressive disorders.

Body System: Psychology

1. A client tries some hallucinogenic medications, and is brought to the emergency room because of a "bad trip". What will this client's treatment most likely include?

   A. Administering lithium
   B. Arm and leg restraints
   C. Seperation from the family
   D. Supportive, repetitive reassurance

2. Identify the medical treatment most often treated with the medication furosemide (Lasix).

   A. Hypotension
   B. Myxedema
   C. Anasarca
   D. Cerebral aneurysm

3. For which medical condition would the nurse expect a 54-year-old client to receive captopril (Capoten)?

   A. Chronic hypertension
   B. Venous thrombosis
   C. Hypertensive crisis
   D. Unstable angina pectoris

1.
Answer: D
Rationale: Will decrease anxiety and promote reality orientation.

Body System: Psychology

2.
Answer: C
Rationale: This is generalized body edema, often treated with diuretics.

Body System: Cardiovascular

3.
Answer: A
Rationale: This is an ACE inhibitor commonly used for chronic hypertension.

Body System: Cardiovascular

1. A client admitted to the hospital in hypertensive crisis is to receive hydralazine (Apresoline) 20 mg IV for a blood pressure greater than 190/100. Choose the best nursing action in response to the physician's order.

   A. Call the physician because the dose is too small
   B. Give the medication as ordered
   C. Give half the dose first to see how it affects the blood pressure
   D. Hold the medication and call the physician because the dose is too large

2. The nurse recognizes that a client who is receiving the medication hydrochlorothiazide (HCTZ) most likely is being treated for which medical condition?

   A. Hypertension
   B. Pulmonary embolism
   C. Increased intercranial pressure
   D. Chronic bronchitis

3. A student working in the ER is asked by the RN to draw up an IV injection of aminocaproic acid (Amicar) for a client. Which condition is the client most likely experiencing?

   A. Hypertensive crisis
   B. Cardiogenic shock
   C. Acute respiratory distress
   D. Hemorrhage

1.
Answer: B
Rationale: Normal dosage range for crisis is 10 - 20 mg.

Body System: Cardiovascular

2.
Answer: A
Rationale: Common use for this diuretic is the control of elevated blood pressure.

Body System: Cardiovascular

3.
Answer: D
Rationale: This medication is used as an antidote to streptokinase, heparin, or can be used with general bleeding disorders like hemophilia.

Body System: Cardiovascular

1. **While admitting a client, the nurse notes allergy to diazepam (Valium). The physician has ordered clonazepam (Klonopin) 1.5 mg PO tid for this client . Which is the best action by the nurse?**

   A.   Give the medication as ordered
   B.   Hold the medication and notify the physician
   C.   Give the medication but monitor the client closely for allergic reactions for four hours
   D.   Give a trial dose of .75 mg and monitor for effect

2. **While assessing a 31-year-old client who is taking haloperidol (Haldol) for hallucinations, the nurse observes that the client is suddenly diaphoretic, extremely rigid, and is unable to speak. Blood pressure was 100/60 a half-hour ago, but now it is 150/70; temperature: 101.2; pulse 126; respiration: 32. All of the following medications are ordered PRN:**

   Acetaminophen (Tylenol) tabs ii for temp > 101 degrees
   Bromocriptine (Parlodel 7.5) mg PO
   Methocarbamol (Robaxin) 2 mg IM
   Notify the physician

   What is the best nursing action at this time?

   A.   Give Tylenol tabs ii and encourage fluids
   B.   Give Robaxin 2mg IM and notify the physician
   C.   Give Tylenol tabs ii, Robaxin 2 gm and notify the physician
   D.   Hold the Haldol, give Parlodel 7.5 mg and notify the physician

1.
Answer: B
Rationale: Klonopin should not be taken if the client is allergic to other benodiazepines such as Valium.

Body System: Neurology

2.
Answer: D
Rationale: The signs and symptoms are of neuroleptic malignant syndrome. It can be reversed if there is early intervention, but it is potentially fatal. Supportive treatment is necessary, but emergency treatment is a dopamine antagonist and a muscle relaxant.

Body System: Neurology

1.   **Identify the situation where the use of terbutaline contraindicated?**

    A.   Transfer of a high-risk labor client to a tertiary facility
    B.   To temporarily stop contractions during fetal distress
    C.   Use as tocolytic therapy in preterm labor
    D.   Prevention of postpartum hemorrhage due to subinvolution

2.   **A pregnant client who is gravida 3, para 2 is admitted with severe pregnancy-induced hypertension. The physician wants to start IV magnesium sulfate at 2 grams per hour. What are the initial side effects the nurse should explain to the client?**

    A.   Hypotension, decreased respirations
    B.   Hypoflexia and flaccid paralysis
    C.   Flushing, sweating, irritability
    D.   Vomiting and diarrhea

1.
Answer: D
Rationale: To stop postpartum bleeding, a medication that increases the contractions of the uterus are needed.

Body System: Obstetric

2.
Answer: C
Rationale: It is common for clients to experience flushing, sweating, and irritability initially with the bolus.

Body System: Obstetric

1.   A client who is at 27 weeks gestation with spontaneously ruptured membranes and no contractions is admitted to the preterm labor unit. Which medication will the nurse most likely administer to promote fetal lung maturation?

       A.   Betamethasone
       B.   Prostaglandin E2
       C.   Magnesium sulfate
       D.   Ritodrine

2.   A postpartum client who has 40 units of Pitocin in her IV bag after the placenta is delivered continues to hemorrhage even after uterine massage. Her vital signs are: pulse 120, blood pressure 90/50, respirations 26. The nurse anticipates the physician will order what medication to stop atony and hemorrhage?

       A.   Ibuprofen
       B.   Prostaglandin F2 alpha
       C.   Ephedrine
       D.   Methergine

3.   A client who has delivered after a 14-hour labor has oxytocin (Pitocin) added to the IV bottle. What is the rationale for giving this medication?

       A.   Prevent uterine atony and hemorrhage
       B.   Decrease milk let-down
       C.   Prolong uterine involution
       D.   Relieve pain

1.
Answer: A
Rationale: Betamethasone is used in two doses to help fetal lung maturity for 26 to 32 week gestation fetuses. These doses are given 24 hours apart, so labor must be delayed for this medication to work.

Body System: Obstetric

2.
Answer: D
Rationale: Methergine is an ergot derivative. Given IV, it will elevate blood pressure and work to contract uterine musculature.

Body System: Obstetric

3.
Answer: A
Rationale: Pitocin post delivery increases uterine contractions to prevent hemorrhage and atony.

Body System: Obstetric

1.   In planning care for a 32-year-old gravida 1, para 0 client who is at 42 weeks gestation and is admitted for induction of labor, the nurse should include what important information about oxytocin (Pitocin) prior to its administration IV?

      A.   IV Pitocin will lower blood pressure

      B.   IV Pitocin is diluted and given as a piggyback

      C.   IV Pitocin has a long half-life

      D.   IV Pitocin is a natural diuretic

2.   When reviewing the product information available on a medication, the nurse finds that it is teratogenic. Which client should not receive this medication?

      A.   Asthmatic

      B.   Pregnant

      C.   Child

      D.   Client with renal failure

3.   Which assessment information best indicates to the nurse that the dose of lithium ordered for a newly diagnosed 22-year-old male client with bipolar disorder is appropriate?

      A.   Appropriate behavior response

      B.   Absence of side effects

      C.   Development of slight weight gain

      D.   Serum blood levels

1.
Answer: B
Rationale: IV Pitocin must always be diluted when given IV as it is caustic to the veins. It is given piggyback in order to stop the medication if needed and still hydrate the client.

Body System: Obstetric

2.
Answer: B
Rationale: The term teratogenic means that the medication may cause abnormal development of the fetus if used during pregnancy. Many medications have not been adequately studied; however, no medication that is known to be teratogenic should be administered to a pregnant client unless the benefits clearly outweigh the risks.

Body System: Obstetric

3.
Answer: D
Rationale: Lithium has a very low margin of safety, which necessitates monitoring blood levels frequently when starting therapy and periodically during therapy. High-risk clients may require daily blood tests. The other choices are not sensitive indicators of therapeutic levels.

Body System: Neurology

1.   The husband of a client who has been taking the tricyclic antide-
       pressant medication imipramine (Trofanil) for three days asks the
       nurse why his wife shows no signs of improvement.   Choose the
       best response by the nurse.

       A.   "The dose is probably too low and will be increased
               gradually until the desired response is seen."
       B.   "Since your wife has not responded after three days, she will
               most likely not get significant relief symptoms from this
               medication and another medication will probably be tried."
       C.   "It usually takes two to four weeks to notice any
               improvement in behavior."
       D.   "It's difficult to assess the level of depression; only your
               wife knows for sure if the medication is working at this
               early stage of therapy."

2.   Which client response indicates to the nurse that the IV amino-
       caproic acid (Amicar) is effective?

       A.   Urine output increases to 45 mL/hour from 22 mL/hour
       B.   Blood pressure increases to 110/66 from 88/42
       C.   Gastric drainage from an NG tube turns a greenish-yellow
               color from bright red
       D.   Serum ammonia level increases from 42 mcg/dl to 55
               mcg/dl

3.   An HIV positive 23-year-old client is beginning a course of treat-
       ment with zidovudine (AZT). Which statement by the client
       indicates to the nurse an understanding of the nurse's instructions
       about the medication?

       A.   "If I am asleep, I can put off taking the medication until I
               wake up because I need rest to keep up my resistance."
       B.   "This medication will cure my HIV in six months to a year."
       C.   "After I have been on this medication for several weeks, I
               can resume my daily routine."
       D.   "If I get a sore throat or fever, I should call the physician."

1.
Answer: C
Rationale: Tricyclic antidepressant medications inhibit reuptake of several   neurotransmitters (norepinephrine, serotonin, and dopamine) in the brain, which may account for their primary action.

Body System: Neurology

2.
Answer: C
Rationale: Amicar is a hemostatic medication that prevents fibrinolysis and stabilizes clot formation. It is an antidote for streptokinase and heparin, and can be used with any severe bleeding disorder like gastric ulcers.

Body System: Cardiovascular

3.
Answer: D
Rationale: These are early signs of infection that may develop into more severe infections in the immune suppressed HIV client.

Body System: Immune

1.   A client develops joint pain and swelling in the great toe of the
        right foot after an eighth treatment with chlorambucil (Leukeran)
        for Hodgkin's disease. Which nursing action is most effective in
        preventing this side effect?

        A.   Ambulate the client the length of the hall tid to promote
                joint mobility
        B.   Encourage the client to drink 2-3 liters of fluid per day
        C.   Administer an ordered PRN dose of acetaminophen
                (Tylenol) 650 mg PO
        D.   Keep the foot of the bed elevated during administration of
                the medication

2.   A client is given methylergonovine maleate (Methergine) 0.2 mg
        by mouth. Which response indicates to the nurse that the medica-
        tion is achieving its desired effect?

        A.   Respiratory rate of 16 breaths per minute
        B.   Blood pressure of 124/78
        C.   Apical pulse of 72 beats per minute
        D.   Uterine fundus firm and in the midline

3.   In planning care for a client with a serum uric acid level of 10.4
        mg/dl, the nurse anticipates teaching the client about the side
        effects of which medication?

        A.   Zidoudine (AZT)
        B.   Probenecid (Benemid)
        C.   Furosemide (Lasix)
        D.   Vincristine (Oncovin)

1.
Answer: B
Rationale: Increasing the fluid intake will help prevent uric acid build-up and eliminate the uric acid from the body.

Body System: Chemotherapy

2.
Answer: D
Rationale: Methergine, an oxytocic class medication, is used postpartum to prevent postpartum hemorrhage due to subinvolution.

Body System: Obstetric

3.
Answer: B
Rationale: Normal uric acid level is 3.5-8.0 mg/dl. It is increased in gout, and Benemid is a commonly used uricosuric agent to lower uric acid levels.

Body System: Analgesic

1. A client with tonic-clonic seizures is to be started on primidone (Mysoline) by mouth. Which medication allergy indicates to the nurse that this medication should be "held" and the physician notified?

    A.   Phenytoin (Dilantin)
    B.   Prochlorperazine (Compazine)
    C.   Phenobarbital (Luminal)
    D.   Propranolol (Inderal)

2. A client asks the nurse what the purpose is to being switched from chlorpromazin (Thorazine) to clozapine (Clozaril). Choose the best answer by the nurse to this question.

    A.   "You are building up a resistance to the Thorzine, so the Clozaril will be more effective".
    B.   "Clorazil produces fewer extrapyramidal reactions than the Thorazine".
    C.   "Your schizophrenia has improved to the point where you no longer need the more potent Thorazine".
    D.   "You better ask your physician since nurses are not allowed to give this information to clients".

3. Which client response best indicates to the nurse that doxepin (Sinequan) is achieving a positive therapeutic effect?

    A.   The client is better able to cope with day-to-day stressors from the environment
    B.   The client reports fewer auditory hallucinations and better thought organization
    C.   The client's blood pressure is now 134/88, down from 162/98 a week ago
    D.   The client displays less paranoid ideation in discussing the illness

1.
Answer: C
Rationale: Primidone is converted into a metabolite form of
                    phenobarbital in the liver — cross allergies are common.

Body System: Neurology

2.
Answer: B
Rationale: Clozaril has fewer extrapyramidal side effects and less
                    incident of tardive dyskinesia, but carries a higher risk of
                    hematologic abnormalities.

Body System: Neurology

3.
Answer: A
Rationale: Doxepin is a tricyclic antidepressant that is also used as an
                    antianxiolytic agent. The goal of therapy is to have the client
                    overcome depression/anxiety and be able to resume normal
                    activities of daily living.

Body System: Neurology

1.   While obtaining the admission assessment and history of a
      55-year-old client, the nurse notes that colchicine 0.6 mg PO is
      being taken each morning. Based on this information, what other
      nursing intervention should be anticipated to be part of the client's
      care?

      A.   Have fluid restrictions of 1000 mL per day
      B.   Be required to ambulate tid the length of the hall
      C.   Receive a purine restricted diet
      D.   Be required to have serum blood levels drawn

2.   Which laboratory value from a client who was taking didanosine
      (ddI, Videx) should be of most concern to the nurse?

      A.   Serum amylase 306 u/l
      B.   Serum SGOT 32 u/l
      C.   WBC 13,000
      D.   Serum potassium 5.2 mEq/l

3.   A 43-year-old client who experiences an acute attack of gout after
      eating "Surf & Turf" at a local steak house is given colchicine 1.2
      mg PO initially, then 0.6 mg q1 hour. At this rate of administra-
      tion, how soon would the maximum cumulative dose of this
      medication be reached?

      A.   4 hours
      B.   6 hours
      C.   9 hours
      D.   10 hours

1.
Answer: C
Rationale: Colchicine is an anti-inflammatory medication used to treat gout. Purines are protein substances found in many meats, fish, meat extracts, etc. that promote uric acid production and make gout worse.

Body System: Gastrointestinal

2.
Answer: A
Rationale: Pancreatitis, a serious side effect of this medication is indicated by a serum amylase 1.5 to 2 times normal (normal=30-170u/l (SI units).

Body System: Immune

3.
Answer: C
Rationale: A total cumulative dose of 6 mg is considered maximum for this medication.

Body System: Gastrointestinal

1.   **A 46-year-old client is taking conjugated estrogen (Premarin) for postmenopausal syndrome. Which reported activity would be of most concern to the clinic nurse?**

    A.   Joining a gourmet cooking club
    B.   Starting to jog two miles per day
    C.   Beginning smoking cigarettes after a four-year abstinence
    D.   Drinking a glass of wine with supper each day

2.   **Which condition is most frequently treated with diphenhydramine (Benadryl)?**

    A.   Relief of allergic reactions
    B.   Relief of chronic angina pain
    C.   Dilation of the bronchioles in asthma
    D.   Stimulation of the cardiac muscles

3.   **A client asks the nurse why the physician prescribed an antihistamine for an upper respiratory viral infection. Which physiological action is expected with this medication?**

    A.   Suppress the CNS and help the client sleep at night
    B.   Decrease the permeability to capillary fluid, thus reducing nasal congestion
    C.   Reduce pain sensation and promote client comfort
    D.   Decrease the production of stomach acid, thereby preventing an ulcer from forming

1.
Answer: C
Rationale: Smoking and estrogen together increase the risk for vascular disease and clot formation.

Body System: Endocrine

2.
Answer: A
Rationale: This is a histamine blocker used for allergic reactions.

Body System: General

3.
Answer: B
Rationale: This is one of the effects of antihistamines.

Body System: Respiratory

1. A hospitalized client with Chronic Obstructive Lung Disease
    (COPD) asks the nurse why the physician will not order diphen-
    hydramine HCL (Benadryl) for nasal congestion. Which response
    by the nurse is most appropriate?

    A.   "Benadryl can cause bronchoconstriction that may make
         your breathing more difficult."
    B.   "Benadryl and theophylline interact in such a way as to
         produce excessive agitation and sleep loss."
    C.   "Because Benadryl tends to dry-up secretions, it may make
         it more difficult for you to cough out your mucus."
    D.   "The physician does not think your congestion is severe
         enough for this medication."

2. A client has just received morphine sulfate, 5 mg IV for chest pain.
    When monitoring side effects, which is the most important?

    A.   Diaphoresis and flushing
    B.   Constipation
    C.   Hypotension
    D.   Suppressed cough reflex

3. Choose the condition most commonly treated with orphenadrine
    citrate (Norgesic).

    A.   Gastroesophageal reflux
    B.   Congestive heart failure
    C.   Back sprain
    D.   Urinary retention

1.
Answer: C
Rationale: Clients with COPD need to remove the secretions from their lungs.

Body System: Respiratory

2.
Answer: C
Rationale: Hypotension may make the client weak or unsteady when getting up causing imbalance or falling.

Body System: Cardiovascular

3.
Answer: C
Rationale: This is a muscle relaxant often used for strains and sprains of major muscles.

Body System: Analgesic

1.   A client, who has been given carbamazepine (Tegretol) for a recently diagnosed seizure disorder, asks the nurse, "How long will I have to be on this medication before it cures me?" Choose the best nursing response.

        A.   "Most clients are cured in 24 to 72 hours."
        B.   "You better ask your physician about that. Nurses can't give out that information."
        C.   "This medication will not cure you, it only controls the symptoms of the disease."
        D.   "It's really hard to say. Every client's response to the medication is very different."

2.   Which condition is most likely to be the reason a child is receiving nystatin (Mycostatin)?

        A.   Viral infection
        B.   Bacterial infection
        C.   Fungal infection
        D.   Nosocomial infection

3.   A client is admitted to the obstetrical unit at 27 weeks gestation with ruptured membranes. In planning care for this client, the nurse anticipates the use of which of the following medication?

        A.   Magnesium sulfate (M_gSO_4)
        B.   Betamethasone
        C.   Exosurf Neonatal
        D.   Ritodrine

1.
Answer: C
Rationale: Anticonvulsant medications only control the seizures; they do not cure the disorder.

Body System: Neurology

2.
Answer: C
Rationale: This is an antifungal medication.

Body System: Antibiotic

3.
Answer: B
Rationale: Betamethasone is a glucocorticoid that will promote the maturation of the fetus' lungs and production of surfactant.

Body System: Obstetric

1.   A physician orders metaproterenol (Alupent) for a client. What route is used to administer this medication?

A.   IV
B.   IM
C.   Inhalation
D.   Rectal suppository

2.   Which side effects will a client most likely experience after receiving a dose of metaproterenol (Alupent)?

A.   Tachycardia, shaking
B.   Bleeding peptic ulcer, vomiting
C.   Moderate hypotension, dizziness
D.   Edema, moon face

3.   The blood level of a client receiving $MgSO_4$ for Pregnancy Induced Hypertension (PIH) is 4.7 mcg/mL. Which nursing intervention is most correct in this situation?

A.   Increase the rate of infusion of the medication
B.   Give calcium gluconate
C.   Begin an infusion of naloxone (Narcan)
D.   Continue the medication at its present rate

1.
Answer: C
Rationale: A potent bronchodilator most often given by hand-held nebulizer (HHN) or respiratory treatments.

Body System: Respiratory

2.
Answer: A
Rationale: This medication stimulates beta receptors to dilate bronchioles, but also stimulates the cardiovascular system.

Body System: Respiratory

3.
Answer: B
Rationale: This blood level is well above the low toxic range of 2. Calcium gluconate is the antidote for $MgSO_4$ toxicity.

Body System: Obstetric

1. **How should a nurse administer ribavirin to a 16-month-old child who has respiratory syncytial virus (RSV)?**

    A. Oral
    B. IM
    C. IV
    D. Aerosol

2. **A client, who is 32 weeks pregnant, is diagnosed with pyelonephritis. What medication would the nurse anticipate the physician prescribing?**

    A. Oxytocin
    B. Magnesium sulfate
    C. Ampicillin
    D. Tetracycline

3. **Which medication is most appropriate to give to a hospitalized alcoholic client who is becoming increasingly irritable and agitated, and displaying tremors of the hands?**

    A. An opiate
    B. A benzodiazepine
    C. A trycyclic antidepressant
    D. A phenothiazine

1.
Answer: D
Rationale: An aerosol particle generator unit aerosolizes this medication for quick absorption by oxygen hood, croup tent or aerosol mask.

Body System: Respiratory

2.
Answer: C
Rationale: This is from the penicillin group and has no known teratogenic effects that may lead to birth defects.

Body System: Antibiotic

3.
Answer: B
Rationale: These medications, such as Librium, have a sedative effect and are often used to control the withdrawal symptoms of alcohol that the client is displaying.

Body System: Neurology

1.   A client who is completing the in-patient segment of a substance
      abuse program was started on disulfiram (Antabuse). Which
      teaching point is most important for the nurse to include in the
      discharge instructions?

      A.   "If you drink alcohol while you are taking this medication,
            you will have nausea, vomiting and elevated blood
            pressure."
      B.   "It is best that this medication be started as late in the
            program as possible."
      C.   "This medication works by desensitizing you to alcohol."
      D.   "You may experience the effects of this medication if you
            drink alcohol as much as two weeks after you stop the
            medication."

2.   A postmenopausal client who has developed major depression is
      started on fluoxetine (Prozac) therapy. Which is the most impor-
      tant point for the nurse to include in the discharge instructions?

      A.   "You can take your daily dose of fluoxetine either in the
            morning or evening."
      B.   "There are no restrictions on driving or other hazardous
            activities because this medication is non-sedating."
      C.   "You may develop a rash or itching when you first start
            taking the medication, but it will go away later."
      D.   "It is safe to take over-the-counter or other prescription
            medications because there are few medication interactions
            with fluoxetine."

3.   Which diet would the nurse anticipate being prescribed for a
      client who recently overdosed on phenelzine sulfate (Nardil)?

      A.   High carbohydrate, low cholesterol
      B.   High protein, high carbohydrate
      C.   Regular, 1 gram sodium
      D.   As tolerated, tyramine-free

1.
Answer: D
Rationale: Disulfiram has a long half life and clients have been known
                   to develop symptoms as much as two weeks after they
                   discontinue the medication.

Body System: Neurology

2.
Answer: C
Rationale: Some of the less serious side effects such as rash and itching
                   occur when first taken, but are easily controlled with
                   antihistamines or corticosteroids.

Body System: Neurology

3.
Answer: D
Rationale: Nardil is a MAO inhibitor, and even though the client may
                   not be currently taking the medication, tyramine foods
                   should be avoided for at least three weeks after the
                   medication is stopped.

Body System: Neurology

1.   A client diagnosed with moderate anxiety is started on a short acting benzodiazepine. Which behavior would be observed in evaluating the effect of this medication?

   A.   Euphoria and restlessness one hour after administration
   B.   Calmer and more controlled after the first 24 hours
   C.   Unsteadiness while ambulating that may lead to falls
   D.   Sleepy and difficult to arouse two hours after administration

2.   A 4-year-old client who has finished a course of chemotherapy for Wilms' Tumor is to receive filgrastim (Neupogen) SC daily for five days. Which response would the nurse note if the filgrastim therapy is effective?

   A.   Decreased immunoglobulin level
   B.   Increased white blood cell count
   C.   Decreased tumor cell levels
   D.   Increased platelet count

3.   A client asks, "Why is the physician prescribing danazol (Danocrine) for my endometriosis?" Select the best response by the nurse.

   A.   Decreases the secretion of FSH and LH
   B.   Increases the production of estrogen
   C.   Causes the body to release an LH surge
   D.   Increases the activity of the ovaries

1.
Answer: B
Rationale: Short acting medications will exert their desired effect within the first 24 hours, sometimes even after the first dose.

Body System: Neurology

2.
Answer: B
Rationale: Neupogen accelerates the maturation and growth of neutrophils that are often decreased by chemotherapy, increasing the WBCs.

Body System: Cardiovascular

3.
Answer: A
Rationale: Danazol is an antigonadotropin that suppresses the production of luteinizing hormone and follicle-stimulating hormone, reducing the engorgement caused in the ectopic endometrial tissue and the accompanying pain.

Body System: Gynecology

1.   **Which client statement indicates the teaching about Graves'
        disease and treatment with I-131 was successful?**

        A.   "For the next three days, I need to drink two to three quarts
                of fluid a day."
        B.   "I can go visit my pregnant sister as soon as I leave here
                today."
        C.   "I shouldn't have any pain or discomfort in my neck."
        D.   "I'll have to stay in the hospital for a few days after you give
                me the medication."

2.   **A client with preterm labor begins to display symptoms of tachy-
        cardia, hypotension, tremors and headache. If she is receiving all
        of the following medications, which one is producing these
        symptoms?**

        A.   Magnesium sulfate
        B.   Nifedipine
        C.   Terbutaline
        D.   Indomethacin

3.   **A client who is in her 30th week of gestation and diagnosed with
        postfetal demise asks the nurse why she is being given a prosta-
        glandin suppository at this time. What nursing response should be
        given to the client?**

        A.   "It will help relieve the pain you will experience when the
                baby is delivered."
        B.   "This will allow you to relax and decrease your anxiety."
        C.   "It will prevent postpartum infections in cases like yours."
        D.   "It will cause labor to start."

1.
Answer: A
Rationale: Extra fluid and good hydration are necessary to purge the body of the radioactive iodine.

Body System: Endocrine

2.
Answer: C
Rationale: These are common side effects of tocolytics like terbutaline. Note the tremors.

Body System: Obstetric

3.
Answer: D
Rationale: Prostaglandin E_2 vaginal suppositories or gel are used to induce labor in cases where there is second or third trimester fetal demise. They stimulate smooth muscle and cause the uterus to contract.

Body System: Obstetric

1.   **Which instruction is most important to give to a client who is receiving sulfamethoxazole (Gantanol)?**

     A.   Chew the tablets completely before swallowing
     B.   Don't be concerned by the blue-colored urine
     C.   Drink 2 to 3 liters of fluid per day
     D.   Call the physician if tinnitus occurs

2.   **In planning care for a client in hypertensive crisis, who is being given nitroprusside (Nipride), the nurse should recognize which response to the medication?**

     A.   Increase in sodium and water excretion
     B.   Prevention of angiotension I from converting to angiotensin II
     C.   Reduction of systemic vascular resistance
     D.   Decreases the contractility of the myocardial fibers

3.   **Which assessments should most concern the nurse who is caring for a client in hypertensive crisis who has been receiving IV nitro-prusside (Nipride) for the past 32 hours?**

     A.   Dilated pupils and pink-colored skin
     B.   Deep, rapid respirations and bounding pulses
     C.   Hyperactive reflexes and loud heart sounds
     D.   Insomnia and mild hypertension

1.
Answer: C
Rationale: Always a good idea to drink extra fluids when on any type of antibiotic. Sulfa medications may cause urinary crystal formation if client is dehydrated.

Body System: Antibiotics

2.
Answer: C
Rationale: Nitroprusside is a member of the nitrate family of medications that causes vasodilation and reduction of after load.

Body System: Cardiovascular

3.
Answer: A
Rationale: These are signs of nitroprusside toxicity, also shallow respirations, weak pulses, suppressed reflexes, distant heart sounds, somnolence, coma and severe hypotension.

Body System: Cardiovascular

1.   A 58-year-old client with chronic bronchitis has two inhalers, one with beclomethasone (Vanceril), the other with metaproterenol (Alupent).   Which instruction is the most appropriate for the nurse to include in the teaching plan for this client?

A.   Use the Vanceril first, followed by the Alupent
B.   Use the Vanceril only in the morning, and the Alupent in the afternoon
C.   Use the Alupent first, followed by the Vanceril
D.   Use the Alupent in the morning, and the Vanceril in the afternoon and evening

2.   Which nursing action would be in order to prevent the development of side effects in a client who was receiving the antibiotic, pentamidine isethionate (Pentam 300)?

A.   Daily weighing to detect fluid retention
B.   Have the client lie down while receiving the medication to prevent hypotension
C.   Keep the client NPO until after the dose is given, then give a calorie-restricted diet
D.   Restrict the client's fluid intake to 1500 mL/24 hours to prevent urinary calculi

1.
Answer: C
Rationale: Metaproterenol (Alupent) is a bronchodilator that opens the
air passages so that the steroid medication (beclomethasone)
can penetrate deeper into the lungs and reduce the
inflammation of the bronchioles and alveoli better.

Body System: Respiratory

2.
Answer: B
Rationale: The two major side effects of this medication are
hypotension and hypoglycemia. Having the client lie down
will prevent falls from postural hypotension.

Body System: Antibiotics

1.   A 44-year-old has been incapacitated with depression for four
        years. The client has had a slight improvement with amitriptyline
        (Elavil); however, the physician decides to prescribe a monoamine
        oxidase inhibitor (MAOI). Identify the most important informa-
        tion to demonstrate understanding by the client.

        A.   Anticholinergic symptoms do not occur with the MAOIs
        B.   Hypertensive crisis may occur if foods high in tyramine
                content are eaten
        C.   MAOIs have few interactions with other medications
        D.   The onset of therapeutic effects is five days

2.   A client is admitted with a low potassium level and is prescribed
        parenteral potassium chloride 40 mEq/L stat. Which method is
        appropriate to administer this dose of potassium?

        A.   Intravenous push
        B.   Concentrated IV infusion
        C.   Diluted IV infusion
        D.   Intramuscularly

3.   Which client statement taking allopurinol (Zyloprim) 300 mg daily
        for treatment of gout indicates the need for additional teaching?

        A.   "Ultraviolet light exposure to my eyes may cause cataracts."
        B.   "I should maintain adequate fluid intake to reduce the
                frequency of attacks."
        C.   "I need to immediately report the development of a rash or
                itching."
        D.   "Medical supervision may be discontinued after
                maintenance dose is prescribed."

1.
Answer: B
Rationale: Hypertensive crisis may follow ingestion of foods that contain tyramine (aged cheese, broad beans, chianti wine, chocolate, pickled herring). The reaction involves a sharp headache, nuchal rigidity, and subarachnoid hemorrhage.

Body System: Neurology

2.
Answer: C
Rationale: Potassium chloride should be diluted with appropriate intravenous solution (usually dextrose) and administered via slow IV infusion. To prevent life-threatening hypokalemia and risk of vascular irritation, never give an intravenous infusion greater than 40 mEq/L in 100 mL.

Body System: General

3.
Answer: D
Rationale: Allopurinol is used for long-term management of gout, and the client should continue medical supervision to monitor for side effects and effectiveness of the medication.

Body System: Analgesic

1.   A nurse is to give **3000 units of heparin, by subcutaneous injection.**
         If the following syringes are available, which one is best for the
         nurse to select for this medication?

         A.   3 mL, 3/8 inch needle
         B.   1 mL, 3/4 inch needle
         C.   1 mL, 5/8 inch needle
         D.   3 mL, 1 inch needle

2.   A physician prescribes metaproterenol (Alupent) by metered dose
         inhalation four times a day for a client with an acute bronchitis.
         Which statement indicates to the nurse that teaching has been
         effective concerning this medication?

         A.   "I need to call the physician immediately if I feel my heart
                  beating fast after using the medicine."
         B.   "I can stop using this when I begin to feel better."
         C.   "I need to hold my breath as long as possible after I take a
                  deep inhalation."
         D.   "I should use this inhaler whenever I get short of breath."

3.   Which measure is appropriate for the nurse to teach a newly
         diagnosed 10-year-old insulin dependent diabetic about self-
         administration of insulin?

         A.   Never use the abdomen as a site because it is very sensitive
                  in a child
         B.   Pinch the skin up to form a subcutaneous pocket
         C.   Do not rub or apply pressure after injection to prevent
                  hematoma formation
         D.   Change the needle after each injection to prevent infection

1.
Answer: C
Rationale: Subcutaneous injections are given into fat pads. A 5/8 inch needle is an adequate length for this purpose. 1 mL syringes are marked in tenths of a mL, which are more accurate for administering small amounts of medication.

Body System: Cardiovascular

2.
Answer: C
Rationale: Holding a breath will help increase the absorption of the medication from the alveoli.

Body System: Respiratory

3.
Answer: B
Rationale: This is the best method for obtaining skin tightness for easy entry of the needle.

Body System: Endocrine

1. Prior to administering methergine to a postpartum client, the nurse assesses the client and finds all of the following symptoms listed below. Which symptom should the nurse be concerned about?

    A.   Lochial flow is increased
    B.   Blood pressure is elevated
    C.   Her face is flushed, skin warm to touch
    D.   She is experiencing uncomfortable afterpains

2. If all of the following medications are available PRN, which should the nurse use for a client who was being detoxified from heroin abuse?

    A.   Narcan
    B.   Naltrexone
    C.   Methadone
    D.   Buprenorphine

3. Which assessment would cause the nurse to suspect that an HIV positive 6-year-old child was developing an adverse reaction to didanosine (ddl; Videx)?

    A.   Mental retardation
    B.   Growth retardation
    C.   Peripheral neuropathy
    D.   Negative nitrogen balance

1.
Answer: B
Rationale: A serious side effect of methergine is hypertension. In clients with elevated blood pressures, another medication should be used.

Body System: Obstetric

2.
Answer: B
Rationale: This is an opioid antagonist that blocks the euphoria produced by heroin. Extended use of naltrexone in conjunction with other treatments produces a loss of interest in heroin.

Body System: Neurology

3.
Answer: C
Rationale: A common and often serious side effect of this medication.

Body System: Antibiotic

1.   When assessing a depressed client who is taking imipramine (Tofranil), what is the nurse's primary concern regarding the effects of this medication?

    A.   Causes liver and renal failure
    B.   Masks the warning signs of an impending suicide
    C.   Must be used in combination with MAO inhibitors
    D.   Elevates mood in 24 to 72 hours

2.   When evaluating a client who is receiving pentamidine isethionate (Pentam 300), what should the nurse expect to see as the client's medical diagnosis?

    A.   Chronic renal failure
    B.   Acquired immune deficiency syndrome
    C.   Diabetes insipidus
    D.   Parkinson's disease

3.   When planning care for a 77-year-old client who is to receive IV lipid emulsions, which action would be priority for safe administration of IV lipid emulsions?

    A.   "Administer at a rate of 10 mL/min."
    B.   "Use tubing that has a filter to prevent emboli."
    C.   "Warm to body temperature prior to administration."
    D.   "Do not piggyback any medications or solutions in with the lipid emulsion."

1.
Answer: B
Rationale: Antidepressants like Tofranil may allow the client to mask the warning signs of suicide and increase their activity level enough to provide them energy to carry out the act.

Body System: Neurology

2.
Answer: B
Rationale: This is a potent antifungal/antiprotazoal medication often used to treat the P. carinii infections that develop secondary to HIV infections.

Body System: Antibiotic

3.
Answer: D
Rationale: No medications or IV solutions should ever be "piggy-backed," or pushed into lipids or hyperalimentation. This increases the risk for infections, and may cause separation or precipitation of the lipids.

Body System: General

1.   **A pregnant client with HIV is in active labor. Which order for the administration of zidovudine (AZT) to this client should the nurse carry out without question?**

   A.   Administer 100 mg q3 hours PO until delivery
   B.   Administer 500 mg IV until crowning, then discontinue
   C.   Administer 2 mg/kg IV over one hour, then continue infusion at 1 mg/kg until umbilical cord is clamped
   D.   Start administering 1 mg/kg IV after the umbilical cord is clamped, and continue for four hours

2.   **Which statement by a client who has a prescription for allopurinol (Zyloprim) 300 mg PO, q 12 hours, would indicate to the nurse that the client requires more teaching concerning this medication?**

   A.   "I should report any rashes, chills or fever to the physician immediately."
   B.   "Drinking alcohol will increase my symptoms."
   C.   "I must avoid over-the-counter medications like ibuprofen and aspirin while I'm taking this medication."
   D.   "If I miss a dose, I should take the dose as soon as I remember."

1.
Answer: C
Rationale: This is the correct protocol to protect the infant from the HIV virus during the labor and delivery process when there is a chance of mixing of blood.

Body System: Immune

2.
Answer: C
Rationale: Client should continue to take NSAID or colchicine during an acute attack of gout because allopurinol helps prevent but does not relieve acute attacks.

Body System: Antibiotic

1. A client who began taking doxepin (Sinequan) 50 mg po qd, seven days ago for an anxiety disorder, complains to the nurse that the medication makes me feel "sleepy and out-of-it" all day long. Select the best response by the nurse.

    A. "Try taking the medication at night before you go to bed."
    B. "Divide the pill in half, and take half in the morning and half in the afternoon."
    C. "We'll talk to the physician about putting you on another medication that won't make you sleepy."
    D. "Tell me why you are so concerned about taking this medication."

2. How should the nurse teach the mother of an anemic 3-year-old child to administer the prescribed liquid ferrous sulfate (Feosol) 3 mL bid?

    A. Offer with 60 cc water
    B. 4 ounces of cold milk
    C. One-half cup orange juice
    D. Any carbonated cola products

3. Which statement best explains the action of edentate calcium disodium (Calcium EDTA) so the parents of a 4 year old with lead poisoning understand what to expect?

    A. Neutralizing the lead in the liver so that it is no longer toxic
    B. Absorbing the lead and eliminating it through the GI tract in the stools
    C. Binding with the lead so that it can be eliminated through the urinary tract
    D. Increasing the metabolism of the lead

1.
Answer: A
Rationale: This is a relatively low dose of this medication and will probably be increased in the future to as much as 300 mg per day. Taking the medication at night does not alter its effects and will help decrease the sedation the client is experiencing during the day.

Body System: Neurology

2.
Answer: C
Rationale: Acidic juices, such as orange or grapefruit, enhance the absorption of iron preparations.

Body System: Gastrointestinal

3.
Answer: C
Rationale: EDTA binds with the lead in the system to produce a substance that can be excreted by the kidneys.

Body System: Gastrointestinal

1. **Prior to becoming pregnant, a 28-year-old client had been taking dicyclomine HCL (Bentyl), a fetal risk category B medication. Which course of action is most appropriate for her when she discovers she is pregnant?**

   A.　Stop taking the medication because it has been demonstrated in tests to cause major birth defects in human fetuses

   B.　Continue taking the medication because human testing has shown no risk for birth defects in human fetuses

   C.　Switch to another medication that has a lower fetal risk category

   D.　Continue taking the medication because it probably is safe, although no human testing has been done, but consult with her physician.

2. **A client diagnosed with genital herpes (HSV-2) is to receive acyclovir (Zovirax) 200 mg PO q4 hours while awake. In developing a teaching plan for this client, the nurse should include which information concerning this medication?**

   A.　If the client has trouble swallowing the pills, they can be crushed or chewed

   B.　If a dose is missed, take twice the dose at the next scheduled time

   C.　Report sore throat, fever or fatigue to the physician

   D.　The infection will be cured after a 7 to 10 day course of treatment

3. **The nurse obtains all of the following information from a client who is to be started on amantadine (Symadine) for treatment of influenza Type A. Which element would cause the most concern in relationship to this medication?**

   A.　Eczematous rash for two weeks

   B.　Client 66 years old

   C.　Type II non-insulin-dependent diabetes

   D.　Parkinson's disease, early stage

1.
Answer: D
Rationale: This statement defines a fetal risk category B medication; always check with the physician when pregnant.

Body System: Gastrointestinal

2.
Answer: C
Rationale: These symptoms may indicate a superinfection that will need treatment quickly.

Body System: Antibiotic

3.
Answer: A
Rationale: This is one of the listed contradictions for taking this medication due to its tendencies to produce rashes.

Body System: Respiratory

1. **Which assessment made by the nurse indicates that the famciclovir (Famvir), which the client has been taking for two weeks, is achieving its desired effects?**

    A. There is a decrease in back pain and arthralgia
    B. There is a decrease in the size and distribution of herpes lesions
    C. The BUN and CrCl indicate normal renal function
    D. The client's HIV viral count is below 100

2. **A client takes oral theophylline medication, and is to be started on a quinolone antibiotic for a respiratory infection. Which interaction can the nurse anticipate from these two medication groups?**

    A. The theophylline medication will increase the serum blood levels of the quinolone antibiotic
    B. Quinolone antibiotics inhibit the effectiveness of theophylline medications
    C. Quinolone antibiotics increase the serum levels of theophylline medications
    D. Theophylline medications block the effects of quinolone antibiotics

3. **A client is to begin taking ciprofloxacin (Cipro) for a Chlamydia trachomatis infection. What information should the nurse include in the teaching plan concerning this medication?**

    A. The medication must be taken with food for best absorption
    B. The client should try to stay in the direct sunlight as much as possible to increase the vitamin D levels to promote healing
    C. If the medication causes GI upset or heart burn, the client should take an antacid
    D. The client should include foods or drinks that have a high source of ascorbic acid

1.
Answer: B
Rationale: This medication is used to treat acute herpes zoster and genital herpes, and successful treatment is indicated by a decrease in the size, pain, itching and spread of the lesions.

Body System: Immune

2.
Answer: C
Rationale: Quinolones reduce hepatic metabolism and increase the serum concentration of theophylline medications.

Body System: Antibiotic

3.
Answer: D
Rationale: Ascorbic acid (vitamin C), along with extra fluid intake, will help prevent crystalluria.

Body System: Antibiotic

1.   **When preparing frozen cryoprecipitate factor VIII for administration to a client with Type A hemophilia, which method is best for the nurse to use to thaw the preparation?**

   A.   Rapidly in the microwave to prevent contamination with bacteria
   B.   At room temperature by placing it in a 37° C bath
   C.   By leaving it in the refrigerator for 24 hours prior to administration
   D.   By placing it in a hot water bath at 45° C

2.   **A client who is taking several medications for hypertension is to be started on colestipol (Colestid) for elevated cholesterol levels. What information is most important for the nurse to include in the teaching plan concerning administration of this medication?**

   A.   The client should decrease intake of fat-soluble vitamins A, D, E, and K to promote maximum colestipol absorption
   B.   The colestipol powder can be taken orally without dilution for quickest effect
   C.   Other medications must be taken one hour before, or four hours after, colestipol
   D.   The client should stop taking the medication if pregnant

3.   **A client taking lovastatin (Mevacor) for high cholesterol levels experiences the following side effects. Which side effect cause should be of most concern?**

   A.   Diarrhea and abdominal bloating
   B.   Headache and dizziness
   C.   Fatigue and weakness
   D.   Clay-colored stools and jaundice

1.
Answer: B
Rationale: Factor VIII should be kept frozen until ready for use.
Thawing at high temperatures can be destructive to Factor
VII activity.

Body System: Cardiovascular

2.
Answer: C
Rationale: Because this medication binds with bile acids in the
intestines, it interferes with the absorption of most
medications if they are taken at the same time as the
colestipol.

Body System: Cardiovascular

3.
Answer: D
Rationale: These may be the first signs of liver failure, the most serious
side effect and complication from this medication. The
other side effects are minor and expected.

Body System: Cardiovascular

1.   A client who was prescribed an albuterol (Proventil, Ventolin) inhaler two days ago returns to the clinic complaining of tremors, anxiety and insomnia. If all the information below was obtained by the nurse during the intake assessment, which behavior would contribute most to the client's complaints?

   A.   Plays bingo nightly in a cigarette smoke-filled room
   B.   Drinks five to eight cups of coffee per day
   C.   Uses the inhaler before meals
   D.   Takes over-the-counter antihistamines for a ragweed allergy

2.   A client is started on cromolyn . Which assessment by the nurse indicates that the medication is achieving its therapeutic response?

   A.   Decreased wheezing and respiratory effort
   B.   Relief of abdominal pain and diarrhea
   C.   Reduction in joint pain and swelling
   D.   Increased urine output and lower blood pressure

3.   What should the recovery room nurse do to avoid diffusion hypoxia in postoperative clients after the administration of nitrous oxide as an anesthetic?

   A.   Keep the head of the bed elevated 35 to 45°
   B.   Assess and maintain the patency of the endotracheal tube
   C.   Administer 100% oxygen for 5 to 10 minutes after the nitrous oxide is stopped
   D.   Encourage the client to cough, turn and deep-breathe every two hours

1.
Answer: B
Rationale: Clients who use adrenergic Beta-2 agonists like albuterol should avoid high intake of caffeine products like chocolate, coffee, tea and colas since they potentiate the effect of the medication.

Body System: Respiratory

2.
Answer: A
Rationale: Cromolyn is used in the treatment of asthma, allergic rhinitis and acute bronchospasms by stabilizing the membranes of sensitized mast cells.

Body System: Respiratory

3.
Answer: C
Rationale: Diffusion hypoxia occurs when the nitrous oxide diffuses rapidly from the blood into the lungs after it is discontinued and dilutes the inspired oxygen concentration to hypoxic levels.

Body System: Respiratory

1. **Which laboratory value indicates to the nurse that a postoperative client was developing a serious complication from halothane that was administered as an anesthetic during a colon resection?**

   A.   Serum potassium 4.9 mEq/l, serum calcium 9.0 mg/dl
   B.   BUN 18 mg/dl, creatinine 1.1 mg/dl
   C.   Thrombocyte count 152,000/mm³
   D.   GGTP 52 IU/dl, total serum bilirubin 10.4 mg/dl

2. **Which physical findings in the health history of a postoperative client would cause the nurse the most concern if thiopental (Pento-thal) was used as the induction anesthesia?**

   A.   History of seizure disorder
   B.   Client age of 78 years
   C.   Long-term moderate hypertension
   D.   History of myxedema

3. **Choose one of the major advantages of using ketamine (Ketalar) as an induction anesthesia over barbiturate agents.**

   A.   The protective airway reflexes remain active with ketamine
   B.   The duration of action of ketamine is much longer than barbiturate medications
   C.   Ketamine is much more potent and lower dosages can be used
   D.   There are fewer side effects, such as nightmares and emergence delirium

1.
Answer: D
Rationale: Halothane has been associated with elevated liver enzymes in postoperative clients due to reduced metabolism in the liver. The condition is called halothane hepatitis. Other values are in normal ranges.

Body System: General

2.
Answer: D
Rationale: Thiopental has been shown to affect thyroid function and should be avoided in clients with a history of thyroid disease.

Body System: Respiratory

3.
Answer: A
Rationale: Clients who receive ketamine maintain their pharyngeal and laryngeal reflexes reducing the possibility of intra- and postoperative aspiration.

Body System: Respiratory

1. A postoperative client with an epidural catheter in place for control of pain complains of a throbbing occipital headache. The nurse assesses the catheter for placement and obtains a good return of cerebrospinal fluid (CSF). Which nursing action is most appropriate at this time?

   A. Give the next scheduled dose of narcotic medication through the epidural catheter as ordered to control the headache

   B. Turn the client on his or her side and carefully reposition the catheter

   C. Hold the next dose of medication and notify the physician

   D. Give the client two acetaminophen (Tylenol) tablets and elevate the head of the bed 45° to help reduce the headache

2. A hospice client with terminal pancreatic cancer is receiving epidural morphine by intermittent injection. Based on the knowledge of the pharmacologic aspects of morphine, the hospice nurse would anticipate which clinical effects when the medication is given by epidural catheter?

   A. Rapid onset of action

   B. Long duration of action

   C. Moderate potency due to dilution in the CSF

   D. Rapid clearance from the CSF

3. The ambulatory surgery nurse would include which teaching points when developing a teaching plan for a client who received a peripheral nerve block with etidocaine (Duranest)?

   A. Avoid sudden position changes for three to five days after surgery

   B. Sleep with the head of the bed flat to prevent hypotension

   C. Protect the area of local anesthesia from trauma for 12 hours after surgery

   D. Maintain a clear liquid diet for 24 hours after surgery

1.
Answer: C
Rationale: Headache, aspiration of CSF along with wet catheter site, paresthesia, motor weakness and bowel or bladder dysfunction are signs of dural procedure and catheter migration. No medication should be given through the catheter until it is repositioned.

Body System: Analgesic

2.
Answer: B
Rationale: Because morphine is more water soluble than lipid soluble, it has a slow onset of action, long duration, high potency, good distribution and slow clearance from the CSF.

Body System: Analgesic

3.
Answer: C
Rationale: Etidocine has a longer duration of action than other types of local anesthetics. Although they average 3 to 6 hour duration, it is not uncommon for them to persist for up to 13 hours after administration.

Body System: Analgesic

1. A client admitted to the medical unit has a serum valproate/valproic acid (Depakene) level drawn with a result of 28 ug/mL. Which is the most appropriate action for the nurse to take at this time?

   A. Place the client on bedrest with bathroom privileges
   B. Institute seizure precautions
   C. Keep the client's room dark and quiet to reduce agitation
   D. Assess the client's blood pressure, pulse and respiratory status

2. In reviewing the medication list of a newly admitted client, the nurse notes that the client takes an anticholinesterase medication. If the client has all of the following conditions, which ones would be treated by this group of medications?

   A. Hypertension and renal failure
   B. Lupus erythematosus and osteoarthritis
   C. Hypothyroidism and adrenal insufficiency
   D. Myasthenia gravis and glaucoma

3. An adult client experiencing an acute myasthenia crisis is to be given pyridostigmine (Mestinon) 25 mg IV bolus. Which nursing precaution is the most important in relation to IV administration of this medication?

   A. Keep a prefilled syringe of 0.1 mg of atropine at the bedside
   B. Connect the client to a bedside ECG monitor
   C. Insert a Foley catheter and monitor urine output hourly
   D. Place an intubation tray and endotracheal tube at the bedside

1.
Answer: B
Rationale: Valproic acid is an anticonvulsant medication. Therapeutic level is 50 to 100 ug/mL. Because this client's level is much lower than therapeutic, he or she would be at high risk for developing seizures.

Body System: Neurology

2.
Answer: D
Rationale: Anticholinesterases (also called cholinesterase inhibitors) are used to treat myasthenia gravis, glaucoma, strabismus, smooth muscle tone and antimuscarinic toxicity.

Body System: General

3.
Answer: A
Rationale: IV administration of pyridostigmine may precipitate a cholinergic crisis. Atropine IV is the antidote for this dangerous condition.

Body System: General

1. A client who has begun using a nicotine transdermal system (Habitrol, Nicoderm) is taking all the following medications. Which interaction should the nurse anticipate for this client?

   A. Decreased absorption of SC NPH insulin
   B. Increased diuretic effects of furosemide (Lasix)
   C. Increased absorption of glutethimide (Doriden)
   D. Increased metabolism of propoxyphene (Darvon)

2. Which point should the nurse include when teaching a client about the use of nicotine resin complex (Nicorette gum)?

   A. It is safe to use during pregnancy
   B. The gum sticks to dentures and dental appliances
   C. Should only chew one piece per hour
   D. Chew gum slowly for 30 minutes but not longer than 45 minutes

3. A psychiatric client taking thioridazine (Mellaril) for schizophrenia develops a sore throat, fever and mouth sores. What is an appropriate action by the nurse in response to these symptoms?

   A. Encourage good oral care four times a day with hydrogen peroxide
   B. Place the client on bedrest and assess blood pressure
   C. Discontinue the medication and obtain a CBC
   D. Place client in seclusion to protect himself and the other clients

1.
Answer: B
Rationale: Client should monitor for signs of dehydration and hypotension while using these two medications at the same time.

Body System: General

2.
Answer: D
Rationale: Chewing slowly for 30 minutes maximizes buccal absorption. After 45 minutes, it is not effective. Other answers are untrue.

Body System: General

3.
Answer: C
Rationale: These symptoms may indicate the development of leukopenia and agranulocytosis, two of the most serious and potentially lethal side effects of antipsychotic medications.

Body System: Neurology

1. The clinic nurse assesses a client who was started on buspirone (BuSpar) two weeks ago for medication effectiveness. What findings indicates that the medication has achieved its therapeutic effects?

    A. Decreased anxiety, restlessness and sleeplessness
    B . Increased alertness and short-term memory
    C. Decrease in joint pain and swelling
    D. Increased urinary output and decreased edema

2. Which statement made by a newly diagnosed Type II diabetic client indicates to the nurse that teaching about glipizide (Glucotrol) had been effective?

    A. "I should avoid drinking all alcohol beverages."
    B. "If I feel sick, I should not take my daily dose of medication."
    C. "It is best if I take the medication with meals."
    D. "I should take the medication before I go to bed for the best effect."

1.
Answer: A
Rationale: Buspirone is an antianxiety agent that inhibits the action of the serotonin. It is used for the short-term management of anxiety disorders.

Body System: Neurology

2.
Answer: A
Rationale: Second generation oral hypoglycemics produce a disulfiram-like reaction in clients who drink alcohol, include nausea, vomiting, headache, hypertension, etc.

Body System: Endocrine

1.   While checking the medication orders on a Type II diabetic client, the nurse notes an order for glyburide (DiaBeta) 50 mg PO each morning. What is the best action for the nurse to take in regard to this order?

   A.   Give the medications, as ordered, because it is the normal dose
   B.   Change the time to "hs", because it is most effective when given at night
   C.   Hold the medication and consult with the physician because the dose is too large
   D.   Give the medication, but consult with the physician, because the dose is too small

2.   A client is started on spironolactone (Aldactone) for treatment of congestive heart failure. Which foods should the nurse instruct the client to avoid while taking this medication?

   A.   Baked chicken and mashed potatoes
   B.   Bananas, salt substitute, and dates
   C.   Chicken and beef liver
   D.   Colas, coffee, and tea

1.
Answer: C
Rationale: Normal dosage range is 5 - 10 mg with a maximum dosage of 20 mg per day.

Body System: Endocrine

2.
Answer: B
Rationale: Spironolactone is a potassium sparing diuretic and foods high in potassium such as fresh fruits, citrus fruits, dried fruits, etc. should not be eaten in large quantities due to the danger of hyperkalemia.

Body System: Cardiovascular

1.   Which laboratory test value indicates that the epoetin alpha
      (Epogen) for a client with chronic renal failure receiving dialysis
      treatments is achieving its therapeutic effects?

      A.   Serum potassium 5.1 mEq/l
      B.   Serum calcium 8.8 mg/dl
      C.   Urine creatinine 3.6 g/24h
      D.   Hemoglobin 15 g/dl

2.   A client taking carisoprodol (Soma) for a work-related back strain
      calls the clinic to tell the nurse of stomach pain when taking the
      medication, so the client stopped taking it yesterday. What
      symptoms should the nurse expect with sudden discontinuation of
      this medication?

      A.   Somnolence and bradycardia
      B.   Headache and nausea
      C.   Hypotension and muscle weakness
      D.   Rash and facial flushing

3.   Which assessments indicates to the nurse that the chlorzoxazone
      (Paraflex) a client has been taking for the past two weeks is
      achieving its therapeutic effects?

      A.   Increased alertness and memory
      B.   Decrease in anxiety and better coping
      C.   Increased circulation to the legs and feet
      D.   Decreased muscle spasms and skeletal pain

1.
Answer: D
Rationale: Epoetin is a synthetic form of erythropoietin that is made in the kidneys and is necessary for red blood cell production. Clients with renal failure no longer make this hormone and become very anemic. If the epoetin is achieving its therapeutic effect, the hemoglobin should increase to normal range (12-18 g/dl).

Body System: Cardiovascular

2.
Answer: B
Rationale: Sudden withdrawal symptoms include insomnia, nausea, headache, spasticity, tachycardia; the medication should be tapered off over one to two weeks.

Body System: Analgesic

3.
Answer: D
Rationale: Chlorozoxazone is classified as a skeletal muscle relaxant and is used to treat the pain and spasms associated with musculoskeletal conditions.

Body System: Analgesic

1.   **What information should the nurse include when developing a teaching plan for a client who has been started on chloroxazone (Paraflex)?**

      A.   Always take the medication with food and/or a full glass of liquid

      B.   Keep the medication in the refrigerator due to its instability

      C.   You can resume normal exercise patterns within 48 hours after starting the medication

      D.   The medication is absorbed best if taken one hour before meals

2.   **A client in the emergency room is to receive a "stat" dose of methocarbamol (Delaxin, Robaxin) 1.5 g IV bolus. Which condition does this client most likely have?**

      A.   Septic shock

      B.   Acute myocardial infarction

      C.   Tetanus

      D.   Kawasaki's syndrome

3.   **What is the most important nursing action when administering IV pancuronium bromide (Pavulon) to a client?**

      A.   Monitor urinary output hourly through a Foley catheter

      B.   Maintain patency of the endotracheal tube and evaluate the function of the positive pressure ventilator

      C.   Keep the head of the bed at 45^0 to prevent aspiration of gastric contents

      D.   Give antiemetic one hour before the medication to suppress the nausea and vomiting often caused when it is given IV

1.
Answer: A
Rationale: GI upset is one of the frequent side effects and can be
decreased by taking the medication with food. The rate of
absorption is not affected by food.

Body System: Analgesic

2.
Answer: C
Rationale: Methocarbamol is a central acting skeletal muscle relaxant
that is used for relief of spasm and pain in musculoskeletal
conditions when given PO or IM. In its IV form, it is used
for relief of the muscle spasms caused by tetanus infection.

Body System: Analgesic

3.
Answer: B
Rationale: Pavulon is a neuromuscular blocker that is used to suppress
skeletal muscle activity during intubation, mechanical
ventilation and surgery. It inactivates all muscle activity in
the body leading to paralysis, including the respiratory
system. Mechanical ventilation is needed to maintain
oxygenation of the tissues.

Body System: Respiratory

1.   **What is the rationale for alternating morphine sulfate and diaze-pam (Valium) IV with IV pancuronium bromide (Pavulon) while a client is connected to a positive pressure ventilator?**

      A.   The morphine and diazepam have the same effects as pancuronium, so less of the medication is needed
      B.   Alternating the medication will decrease the side effects of each individual medication
      C.   Pancuronium only paralyzes the muscles, but does not affect the client's level of consciousness or pain response
      D.   The medications potentiate each other and makes them more effective than if given alone

2.   **Which laboratory value indicates that the client is developing a serious complication secondary to therapy with methotrexate (Folex PFS)?**

      A.   Serum potassium 2.1 mEq/l
      B.   Platelet count 92,000/mm^3
      C.   Urine creatinine 0.6 g/24h
      D.   White blood cell count 9,200/mm^3

3.   **The nurse instructs the client who started methotrexate (Folex PFS) for treatment of severe rheumatoid arthritis to avoid which foods?**

      A.   Cola, coffee and tea
      B.   Oranges, bananas and raisins
      C.   Broccoli, cabbage and cauliflower
      D.   Organ meats, dried beans and shell fish

1.
Answer: C
Rationale: Clients receiving pancuronium only will remain wide awake and alert, but without the ability to move or breathe; a very frightening situation. Diazepam induces sleep, and has an amnesic effect; morphine relieves pain, induces sleep, and alters the perception of stimuli.

Body System: Respiratory

2.
Answer: B
Rationale: Normal platelet count is 150,000 to 400,000. A value below 100,000 indicates the development of thrombocytopenia, a serious condition that may lead to uncontrolled bleeding and death.

Body System: Chemotherapy

3.
Answer: D
Rationale: Clients receiving this medication should be on a low purine diet (like the diet for clients with gout) because of the tendency for elevated uric acid levels.

Body System: Chemotherapy

1.   **Which statement by a client with HIV indicates understanding the nurse's instructions concerning zidovudine (Retrovir)?**

   A.   "I need to take this medication to prevent nausea."
   B.   "If I develop a bad headache or my feet swell, I should skip a dose."
   C.   "I should take the medication one hour before meals."
   D.   "I can expect improvement in my condition within one week."

2.   **Which common side effects would the nurse expect when the client has been receiving zalcitabine (Hivid) for one month?**

   A.   Oral lesions and impaired swallowing ability
   B.   Elevated serum potassium levels
   C.   Decreased blood pressure and bradycardia
   D.   Decreased blood sugar levels

3.   **What condition would be suspected if an HIV client has a decrease in the CD4 count and is started on pentamidine (Nebupent, Pentam 300)?**

   A.   Kaposi's sarcoma
   B.   *Pneumocystis carinii* pneumonia
   C.   Cytomegalovirus
   D.   Low CD+ count

1.
Answer: C
Rationale: If the medication is taken with a high fat meal, the time of peak serum level is delayed and reduces the effectiveness of the medication.

Body System: Immune

2.
Answer: A
Rationale: Oral lesions and swelling in the pharynx are common side effects of this medication and should be assessed on a weekly basis.

Body System: Immune

3.
Answer: B
Rationale: Pentamidine is a potent antifungal medication and one of the few that has any success in treating this infection.

Body System: Immune

1.　　　Which physical response indicates to the nurse that the ganciclovir sodium (Cytovene) prescribed for an HIV client with opportunistic cytomegalovirus retinitis was producing a serious side effect?

    A.　　　Orange-colored urine and skin
    B.　　　Elevated calcium and potassium levels
    C.　　　Decrease in RBC count and hemoglobin
    D.　　　Hypoglycemia and frequent PVCs

2.　　　How should the nurse administer IV furosemide?

    A.　　　Slowly at 1 to 2 minutes per mL
    B.　　　IV piggyback to prevent hypotension
    C.　　　Quickly by IV push
    D.　　　Through a deep vein catheter

3.　　　Choose the best course of action to be taken by the nurse for a client who has developed orthostatic hypotension following the administration of furosemide.

    A.　　　Start IV fluids
    B.　　　Start vasopressor agents
    C.　　　Insert an indwelling (Foley) catheter
    D.　　　Assist with position changes

1.
Answer: C
Rationale: One of the most serious side effects of ganciclovir is bone marrow depression and aplastic anemia that may lead to death.

Body System: Immune

2.
Answer: A
Rationale: Furosemide is given at a rate of 1 cc per minute IV.

Body System: Cardiovascular

3.
Answer: D
Rationale: Orthostatic hypotension is a safety issue, so assistance is necessary.

Body System: Cardiovascular

1. **What is the most important nursing consideration when giving aspirin to a client?**

    A.   Always give the medication before the pain starts
    B.   Monitor for effectiveness
    C.   Give with a full glass of water or food
    D.   Never give IM injections due to bleeding tendencies

2. **Identify some early signs that could indicate lanoxin (Digoxin) toxicity.**

    A.   Bradycardia, AV block
    B.   Blurred vision; ventricular tachycardia
    C.   Renal failure; aplastic anemia
    D.   Disorientation; vomiting

3. **What information should be included when teaching a female client about the metabolic effects of conjugated estrogen (Premarin)?**

    A.   Reduces blood cholesterol and protein synthesis
    B.   Decreases sodium and water retention
    C.   Decreases the production of oils from the sebaceous glands
    D.   Increases mild production postpartum

1.
Answer: C
Rationale: Gastric irritation, a major side effect of ASA, can be prevented if taken with food or liquid.

Body System: General

2.
Answer: D
Rationale: These along with GI upset are early signs

Body System: Cardiovascular

3.
Answer: A
Rationale: These are two of the common metabolic effects of this medication.

Body System: Endocrine

1.   **Which phrase best explains the medication, Micronase, to a newly diagnosed Type II diabetic?**

   A.   Increases the insulin secretions of the pancreas
   B.   Blocks insulin absorption in the cells
   C.   Reduces the breakdown of the insulin in the blood
   D.   Replaces insulin your body does not make

2.   **Which statement is most appropriate for the nurse to include in the discharge instructions for a client who has a prescription for naproxen (Naprosyn)?**

   A.   "Make sure you take the medication with food or meals."
   B.   "Limit your intake of foods containing potassium, such as citrus, bananas, meats, etc."
   C.   "You must drink 2-3 liters of fluid each day while taking this medication."
   D.   "Eat no more than 2 grams of sodium each day to prevent edema."

1.
Answer: A
Rationale: This is a second generation antiabetic medication that
lowers the blood sugar by stimulating the pancreas to
increase its levels of insulin production.

Body System: Endocrine

2.
Answer: A
Rationale: Can cause gastritis or ulcers if taken on an empty stomach.

Body System: Analgesic

DRUG CLASSES
PSYCHOTROPIC DRUGS

Sedating drugs including:
* Anti-anxiety drugs/sleep aids (Benzodiazepines such as aprazolam/Xanax, diazepam/Valium, flurazepam/Dalmane, etc.)
* Hypnotics (temazepam/Restoril, triazolam/Halcion, etc.)
* Barbituates (phenobarbital, butabarbital, secobarbital, etc.)
* Most common side effects are drowsiness; patients should be advised not to drive or operate machinery while using these drugs
* Most have habituating/addictive properties
* Are intended for short term use only

Antidepressants including:
* Tricyclic antidepressants (amitriptyline/Elavil, imipramine/Tofranil, etc.)
* May cause cardiac dysrhythmias, may be deadly if overdose, cause drowsiness
* SSRIs/Selective Serotonin Reuptake Inhibitors(fluoxitine/Prozac, paroxetine/Paxil, sertraline/Zoloft
* Fluoxitine/Prozac may cause agitation, nightmares, and sertraline/ Zoloft may cause sleepiness
* MAOIs/Monamine Oxidase Inhibitors(tranylcypromine/Parnate and phenetzine/Nardil)
* MAOIs require dietary modifications. No tyramine which is found in aged or fermented foods such as aged cheese, wine, smoked meats or fish, yeast. These foods must be avoided. Questions about foods to be avoided are quite often on NCLEX.
* Lithium carbonate is used for bipolar disorder. Monitor drug levels
* Signs of lithium toxicity include drowsiness, slurred speech, seizures, hypotension. Toxic levels are those above 2-2.5 mEq/L. "Levels above 2 are too much"

Antipsychotics including:
* Haloperidol/Haldol
* Phenothiazines (chlorpramzine/Thorazine, fluphenazine/Prolixin)

OTHER NEUROLOGIC AGENTS

Antiseizure drugs including:
* Phenytoin/Dilantin. Monitor blood levels. May cause gingival hyperplasia
* Phenobarbital
* Valproic acid
* Depakote

CARDIOVASCULAR AGENTS

Antihypertensives including:
* Diuretics including loop diuretics (furosemide/Lasix) thiazide diuretics (hydrochlorathiazied/Diuril), potassium sparing diuretics (spironolactone/Aldactone)
* Watch for dehydration, hypokalemia (low potassium) with loop diuretics particularly and sometimes thiazide diuretics
* Calcium channel blockers including dilatiazem/Cardizem, verapamil/Calan
* Angiotenson Converting Enzyme Inhibitors/ACE inhibitors (enalapril/Vasotec, captopril/Capoten)
* Beta Blockers (propanolol/Inderal, metoprolol/Lopressor, atenolol/Tenormin)
* Alpha blockers (praxosin/Minipress)
 Drugs for heart failure including:
* Digitalis/Lanoxin usually on exam
* With digitalis monitor for toxicity as evidenced by dysrhythmias, nausea, headache, yellow/green vision
* If given with diuretic, hypokalemia puts patient at high risk for toxicity
* Diuretics, as listed above

Anticoagulants including:
* Heparin-given subcutaneously only usually in abdomen
* Warfarin/Coumadin takes 4-7 days to reach full potency
* Monitor clotting times

* Patients must not take aspirin or NSAIDs (non-steroidal anti-inflammatory drugs such as ibuprofen or naprosyn). Will cause more risk of bleeding
* Bruising common. Should wear Med-Alert bracelet

Anti-lipid agents including:
* Statins such as atorvastatin/lipitor, lovastatin/Mevacor: need to monitor liver function
* Bile acid sequestrants such as clofibrate/Questran
* Nicotinic acid: may cause severe flushing

Dysrhythmias including:
* Lidocaine
* Beta blockers or calcium channel blockers
Antianginal agents including:
* Nitrogycerine
* May be given for chest pain sublingually, one tab every 5 minutes x 3, then call 911 if chest pain persists
* Keep NTG dry and on person, replace every 6 months
* Isobidide/Isordil

GASTROINTESTINAL DRUGS

Antacids over the counter including:
* Mylanta
* Riopan
* Gelusil

H2 antagonists(blocks about 70% of stomach acid)
* Cimetadine/Tagamet
* Ranitadine/Zantac
* Famotidine/Pepcid
* Nizatidine/Axid
Proton Pump inhibitors(block up to 100% of stomach acid):
* Omeprazole/Prilosec
* Prevacid

RESPIRATORY DRUGS

Antihistamines including:
* Sedating drugs such as diphenhydromine/Benadryl
* Non-sedating drugs such as Claritin, Allegra, Zyrtec

Decongestants including:
* Pseudoephedrine/Sudafed

Inhalers including:
* Steroid inhalers fluticonazone/Flovent, Azmacort
* Bronchodilator inhalers albuterol/Proventil

Cough medicines including:
* Dextromethorophan/Robitussin DM
* Glyceryl guiacolate/Robitussin plain

Bronchodilators including:
* Albuterol/Proventil
* Theophylline/Theo-Dur-monitor blood levels
* May cause jitteriness, cardiac dysrhythmias

ANTIBIOTICS

Penicillins including:
* Amoxil/Amoxicillin * Pen VK * Procaine penicillin * Penicillin is number one drug allergy * If allergic to penicillin, may use erythromycin

Macrolides including:
* Erythromycin/Ery-tab * Clarithromycin/Biaxin * Azithromycin/Zithromax
Cephalosporins including: * Cefaclor/Ceclor * Cephalexin/Keflex * Cefzil * Cefuroxime/Rocephin-given IM

Quinolones including:
* Ciprofloxin/Cipro * Floxin * Levaquin * Tequin * Not to be used in children

Tetracyclines including:
* Doxycycline/Vibramycin * Minocin * May cause darkened teeth in babies if mother takes during pregnancy * Take 1 hour before or 2 hours after meals. Avoid sun

Antifungals including:
* Nystatin/Mycostatin * Nizoral, Lamisil * Flagyl-alcohol will make very nauseous if taken with Flagyl

ENDOCRINE DRUGS

Thyroid medications-levothyroxine/Synthroid Medications for Type II Diabetes including:
* Biguianides/Glucophage * Sulfonamides/Glucotrol, glypizide * Insulin sensitizing agents-Avandia

Insulins including:
* Regular/short acting-onset 1/2-1 hour * NPH/intermediate acting-onset 1-3 hours * Long acting-onset 4-6 hours * Given subcutaneously

Steroids including:
* Prednisone/Decadron * Prednisone/Medrol * Cortisone * All have anti-inflammatory, anti-immune properties * Multiple side effects including altered immune system, mood changes, buffalo hump, moon face, acne, hirsutism, striae, risk of infection, fluid retention, hypertension

ANALGESICS NSAIDs-Non-steroidal anti-inflammatories including:
* Naprosyn/Aleve, Ansaid * Ibuprofen/Rufen, Advil, Motrin * Aspirin * All have anti-pyretic/fever reducing properties * May cause problems with platelet function, not to be used with clotting disorders Acetominphen/Tylenol-fever reducer, analgesic * High doses may lead to liver damage

Narcotic pain relievers including
* Hydrocodone/Lortab * Codeine/Tylenol #3 * Meperidine/Demerol * Morphine